W0107384

H.-P. Breuel · Clinical Pharmacology in the Elderly

Springer-Verlag Berlin Heidelberg GmbH

H.-P. Breuel

Clinical Pharmacology in the Elderly

Reference Ranges and Biological Variations
After Repeated Measurements

With contributions by
P.R. Heine, J. Horkulak, and G. Weyer

Preface by Prof. Dr. Jochen Kuhlmann

With 5 Figures and 201 Tables

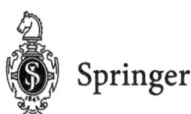 Springer

Prof. Dr. Hans-Peter Breuel
Pharmacon Research
Gesellschaft für Arzneimittelforschung mbH
Carmerstrasse 2
10623 Berlin
Germany

ISBN 978-3-540-59495-6

Library of Congress Cataloging-in-Publication Data. H.-P. Breuel: Clinical Pharmacology in the Elderly. Reference Ranges and Biological Variations After Repeated Measurements. p. cm. Includes bibliographical references. ISBN 3-540-59495-7 (alk. paper) 1. Geriatrics, Gerontology. QGR367.P38 1996 616.7'25077-dc20 DNLM/DDLC for Library of Congress 95-9938 CIP

ISBN 978-3-540-59495-6   ISBN 978-3-642-60998-5 (eBook)
DOI 10.1007/978-3-642-60998-5

© Springer-Verlag Berlin Heidelberg 1996
Originally published by Springer-Verlag Berlin Heidelberg New York in 1996

Typesetting: Text & Grafik, Heidelberg

SPIN: 10499243   27/3136 – Printed on acid free paper

Preface

The appropriate and rational use of drugs by the elderly is a matter of growing medical and social concern. Persons aged 65 years and older constitute about 12%—15% of the population in the Western world, and the total number of the elderly will increase significantly in the coming years. This population accounts for 30% of all the prescription drugs used.

Aging, specifically the transition from middle to old age, is a complex process. From the perspective of clinical pharmacology, these pathophysiological changes may reasonably be expected to alter responsiveness to drugs. The age-related differences in response to drugs can arise from alterations in pharmacokinetics or pharmacodynamics. This makes it mandatory that clinical pharmacological studies be carried out in the elderly during extended phase I studies. The older the population likely to use the drug, the more important it is to include the very old. It is also important not to exclude unnecessarily patients with concomitant illnesses; it is only by observing such patients that drug—disease interactions can be detected.

Reports from surveillance systems have greatly increased our awareness of problems associated with drug therapy in old age. However, there are few publications that present reference ranges for elderly subjects, and, with the exception of renally excreted drugs, present data are insufficient to make recommendations regarding doses of drugs in the elderly. The guideline "Studies in Support of Special Populations: Geriatrics," prepared by the International Conference on Harmonization (ICH), calls for early pharmacokinetic studies, investigation of possible age-related differences in end-organ responses, conducting appropriate drug interaction studies, and including the elderly in phase II and III studies and assessing the results for age-associated effects on efficacy and safety. The inclusion of elderly subjects in controlled clinical trials includes complex methodological concerns such as experimental design, sample size, control groups, subject inclusion and exclusion criteria, drop-out rules, and the choice of appropriate outcome measurements. In turn, these factors determine the proper statistical methods to be applied in analyzing the results.

This book opens with theories of aging and gives an overview of published data on changes of body functions, especially changes in the central nervous system, cardiovascular and pulmonary changes, changes in clinical chemistry and hematology, and changes in pharmacokinetics and receptor sensitivity among young and elderly subjects, including geriatric patients. Chapter 4 focuses on practical aspects in performing clinical trials in elderly subjects. The major part of this volume presents experimental findings from more than 2500 healthy young and elderly subjects (aged 20—39 and 50—80 years). The data originate from subjects who participated in phase I studies performed by the authors as principal investigators. The studies had virtually uniform inclusion and exclusion criteria, and all examinations were performed using the same technical methods.

This volume contains the most comprehensive data on young and elderly healthy subjects that have been published. The numerous data on blood pressure monitoring, ECG, spirometry, clinical chemical laboratory, hematology, and adverse events provide a good basis for evaluating trends and a global overview of changes with age. It is hoped that this book will find its way into the libraries of all physicians interested and involved in clinicopharmacological trials as an excellent reference book.

Prof. Dr. JOCHEN KUHLMANN
Institute for Clinical Pharmacology
International BAYER AG
Wuppertal, Germany

Contents

1 Introduction

Clinical pharmacological studies — the first steps in the clinical development of new chemical entities or new pharmaceutical forms of marketed substances — are performed primarily in young healthy subjects, typically in those aged 18 to 30 years. However, as the elderly proportion of the population increases in all industrial countries, there is a great likelihood that a drug is prescribed often, if not solely, to older patients. Moreover, the incidence of diseases and disorders that require treatment is known to increase with age (Rogers and Spector 1984; Grahame-Smith and Aronson 1984).

Therefore, elderly subjects are now generally included in phases II and III of the clinical development of new drugs, during which at least some aspects of treatment in this large patient group are covered. However, it is obviously important that the clinical pharmacological profile of a new drug should be studied thoroughly before applying it to any particular cohort, particularly as medical surveillance becomes less intensive in the later stages of clinical development (e.g., ambulatory rather than in-house). Moreover, the elderly respond differently to drugs than do younger people (Lamy 1991): their physiological response to drugs is much more scattered, and the predictability of drug action is much less certain (Lamy 1986). Hence, it is now common practice to conduct select phase I studies in elderly subjects, either at the end of the phase I program or parallel to phase II development, when evidence has been presented of the drug's efficacy in young subjects.

At this point it is appropriate to ask what is meant by "the elderly." Clinical pharmacological guidelines such as the Guideline for the Study of Drugs Likely to be Used in the Elderly (FDA 1989) and textbook recommendations (Spilker 1986) often refer to the elderly as those aged 65 years or older. While gerontologists take a more differentiated view (Levinson et al. 1978; Santrock 1985) and distinguish between (a) close of middle adulthood (50 to 59 years), (b) late adult transition (60 to 65 years), and (c) late adulthood (over 65 years), even such a classification has only limited value for a general categorization of aging, considering the large variability of adult development and ongoing aging processes, and considering that it is impossible to distinguish between normal aging and secondary changes due to diseases and/or destructive life-style habits. Indeed, aging must be regarded as a highly individualized process that cannot be defined by chronological landmarks.

Clinical and clinical pharmacological studies of the age dependency of various biological parameters (see Chap. 3 for an overview) all show that the relevant aging processes begin between the ages of 50 and 60 years, followed by a fairly rapid decline in body functions (Rowe and Troen 1980). Therefore, if a chronological distinction can be made at all, the age limit for clinical pharmacological studies in the elderly should be lower than 65 years. There are both ethical and methodological aspects to consider here: the transition from "healthy" to "ill" is fluid in the elderly, and there is a higher probability that inapparent concomitant diseases become manifest under stress. The prevalence of autopsy-documented diseases is higher than the prevalence of clinically apparent diseases (Tejada et al. 1968; Kennedy et al. 1977). Yet clinically inapparent diseases can go undiscovered after a routine screening based on history, physical examination, resting ECG, and blood chemistry parameters. Furthermore, considering that participation in a clinical trial is a stress factor that could have a negative impact on a subject's compensatory mechanisms, which even at the beginning of the aging process are already in decline, the risk of severe adverse events is bound to increase with age (e.g., decrease in myocardial oxygen supply), even if these are not immediately manifest at the close of a clinical study. In addition, there is a danger that a study in the very elderly describes less the fundamental influence of defined aging processes on a drug's clinical pharmacological profile than a series of individual observations with great variability, thus making it very difficult to draw general conclusions.

When designing and interpreting phase I studies in the elderly, which are mainly designed as cross-sectional trials, i.e., a comparison of two or more age groups, it is important to remember that subjects older than 75 years represent a sample of biologically superior survivors from a cohort that has experienced at least 75% mortality (Rowe and Troen 1980), and that these subjects can show findings that are not related to aging per se but rather to a progressive loss of individuals with high risk values ("selective mortality").

By their very nature, clinical pharmacological trials are comparative studies: a comparison is made of data with and without medication, and between recorded values and the norm, i.e., reference ranges of the normal population. The problems associated with reference ranges have been dealt with extensively elsewhere (Harris 1988; Fraser et al. 1989a; Trowbridge et al. 1989; Boyd and Lacher 1982; Gräsbeck and Ahlström 1981); however, it must be said that they remain indispensable in clinical pharmacological studies for inclusion and exclusion of study participants and for interpreting study results, especially in studies with small sample sizes and for analysis of repeated measurements.

There are few publications that present reference ranges for elderly subjects. In particular, there are scarcely any data that meet the specific needs of clinical pharmacology (healthy subjects, exclusion of comedication and codiseases, defined inclusion and exclusion criteria). And there are very few data on repeated measurements from elderly and young healthy subjects in clinical pharmacological studies. The data presented below are therefore intended as a contribution to solving this problem.

2 Theories of Aging

The modern biological theories of aging can be grouped as presented below.

Genome or Genetic Aging Theory Groups. The genetic aging theory is based on the belief that genes are programmed for aging and/or death of an organism (Hayflick 1961, 1975; Medvedev 1972; Roth 1980) with nonmodifiable boundaries for the duration of life.

Physiological Theories. The most widely accepted of the physiological theories of aging is the cross-link or collagen theory (Bjorksten 1971; Ebersole and Hess 1990), which points to the importance of time-related changes in the extra-cellular protein matrix. Chemical reactions create strong bands between molecular structures that are normally separate (cross-linking). Cross-linking produces irreparable damage to DNA and thus causes cell death. Collagen and elastin are important indicators that cross-linking has occurred, leading to changes in connective tissue with typical age-related effects on the heart, lung, arteries, and other organs. The waste product theory (Davies 1985; Sohal and Allen 1985), another physiological theory of aging, attributes aging to an accumulation of waste products such as lipofuscin, as an endproduct of lipid peroxidation induced by free radicals, and posits a link between oxygen consumption, free radicals, lipofuscin, and aging.

Immunological Theory. The immunological theory (Schimke 1980; Lakatta and Yin 1982) maintains that aging is an autoimmune process, as a consequence of which the immune system fails to recognize its own cells, thus causing cell destruction or cell death.

None of these theories can alone explain the very different and at times very specific aging processes in the various organ systems, but they permit a logical classification of some aspects of aging.

3 Changes in Body Functions, Pharmacokinetics, and Receptor Sensitivity with Age

3.1 Changes in Central Nervous System

Aging involves many different phenomena, among them changes in the structure and function of the central nervous system (CNS). Structural changes can be observed on the molecular and cellular levels as well as in the gross morphological appearance of the brain. Changes in CNS function can also be studied on different assessment levels, ranging from biochemical studies of nerve cell metabolism through neurophysiological measurements of electro-cortical activity and psychometric assessments of behavior.

When evaluating the effects of centrally acting drugs in elderly healthy volunteers, it is important to know what particular characteristics of this group differ in what way from young subjects or from geriatric patients. The following summarizes some of the most typical phenomena of normal aging. However, when describing age-related changes in CNS structure and function, it should be recognized that the differences between age groups may be smaller than the differences within one age group. The range of interindividual variability includes also the absence of any age-related changes in some individuals in some of the variables under consideration.

3.1.1 Brain Structure and Function

Aging of the human CNS typically involves a shrinkage of the brain, which becomes visible with imaging techniques as computed tomography or in autopsy by a narrowing of brain gyri, an inverse widening of brain sulci, and an increase in the size of brain ventricles. The decrease in brain volume and brain weight is due to neuronal atrophy and neuronal loss. Atrophic processes that result in neuronal loss are not distributed homogeneously over the different regions of the brain. The decrease in the numbers of neurons is apparently greater in the temporal and frontal cortex than in the diencephalon, cerebellum, and brainstem (Critchley 1942). Among the cortical areas that appear to be most affected by neuronal atrophy are the superior temporal gyrus, precentral gyrus, and area striata, whereas the adjacent areas of the inferior temporal gyrus and postcentral gyrus do not show a comparable loss of nerve cells (Brody 1973). The amount of decrement in the weight of the brain that can be attributed to normal aging has been estimated to be in the order of 5%–8% (Ferszt and Gertz 1982).

There is some indication that the atrophic processes may be associated with decreases in cerebral blood flow (Melamed et al. 1980) and with cerebral oxygen and glucose utilization (Frackowiak et al. 1980). This is particularly true in dementia, whereas the evidence is inconsistent in normal aging. More recent studies in normal older subjects using positron emmission tomography techniques have failed to reveal age-correlated changes in these parameters of brain metabolism (e.g., DeLeon et al. 1983; Rapoport et al. 1983). Thus it is difficult to ascertain whether changes in cerebral metabolism constitute normal concomitants of aging, systematically related to changes in brain structure, or whether the relationship between changes in brain structure and function is due to pathological processes.

The question is also unresolved with regard to the various age-related changes that have been studied on the cellular level, for example, decreases in the amount of cytoplasmic RNA and in the activity of cytoplasmic enzymes and neuronal organelles. All these cellular events can result from changes in the extraneuronal environment or from changes in neuronal structure or cellular biochemistry (Bondareff 1977).

The intraneuronal accumulation of lipofuscin pigment is one of the phenomena that appears to be primarily associated with chronological age (Brizzee et al. 1974). However, its relation to neuronal function is not known. Intraneuronal fibrillary tangles and so-called senile plaques, on the other hand, are commonly found in the brains of demented patients and only to a far lesser extent in the brains of clinically inconspicuous older subjects. The occurrence of fibrillary tangles and plaques seems to be the result of pathological processes and not primarily related to chronological age (Tomlinson et al. 1968; Tomlinson 1982).

One consistent finding of age-related changes in interneuronal connections in the CNS is the postsynaptic decrease in the density of α- and β-adrenergic and dopaminergic receptors. However, effects of this on any specific physiological functions have not been documented in healthy elderly adults (Palm and Wiemer 1982).

The central cholinergic deficit that is well documented for patients suffering from dementia of the Alzheimer type (Davies 1979; Kopelman 1986; Perry et al. 1977) seems to be specific to the pathophysiology of this disease and is not found in normal aging.

3.1.2 Electroencephalogram

The electroencephalogram (EEG) is the traditional and most popular measure of cortical function. The resting EEG of older individuals typically shows a slowing of the dominant alpha frequency (8–13 Hz), an increase in diffuse slow-wave activity that consists of delta (1–3 Hz) and theta (4–7 Hz) waves appearing in various recording sites on the head, and focal changes located predominantly in the left temporal region (Christian 1984; Matejcek 1984; Obrist 1979).

The average alpha frequency decreases rather linearly with age from 10–10.5 Hz in young adults to 8.5–9 Hz in 80-year-old mentally healthy individuals. At the same time there is a decline in the amplitude of alpha waves and a decrease in alpha percentage time of the record. In demented patients the average alpha frequency may be even lower than 7 Hz, but a relationship between alpha slowing and cognitive function has not been found within the normal range.

Diffuse slow-wave activity is seen in an increasing proportion of the population as age increases. The degree of diffuse EEG slowing has been found to be related to the degree of cognitive deterioration in psychiatric patients (Duffy et al. 1984; McAdam and Robinson 1956). However, as with alpha slowing, this correlation is not seen in elderly healthy volunteers (Wang and Busse 1969).

Focal slow-wave activity is seen in about 30%–50% of nonpatient subjects over 60 years of age as compared with 3%–4% in 20- to 30-year-old individuals (Busse et al. 1954). The appearance of this EEG phenomenon, consisting of episodic bursts of high voltage slow waves from a small region, does not seem to be related to measures of cognitive function.

Suggestive explanations of the slowing of the EEG with age rely on the reduced blood supply, neuronal loss, and reduced metabolic needs of the aged brain (Obrist 1979). However, direct evidence for this is not available.

Fast EEG activity above the alpha frequency band, i.e., beta waves (14–30 Hz and above) is seen most frequently in periods of arousal and mental activity. It appears only occasionally in the resting EEG. The presence of beta activity in the resting EEG has been reported to increase with age up to about 60–70 years and to decrease again beyond this age (Busse et al. 1956; Gibbs and Gibbs 1950; Roubicek and Roth 1967). Severely deteriorated psychiatric patients exhibit less beta activity — if any — than normal elderly subjects (Barnes et al. 1956; Mundy-Castle et al. 1954). In normal volunteers aged 85 years and above a relationship has been found between the proportion of beta activity and cognitive performance and self-report measures of well-being (Weidenhammer and Engel 1988).

In addition to the age-related changes in the spontaneous resting EEG, there are also characteristic alterations in electrocortical measures of reactivity to external stimulation and internal events. Elderly subjects are less responsive to simple sensory stimuli as well as to more complex events requiring focused attention or cognitive processing. This can be seen, for example, in the alpha blocking response, which may be less complete than in the young, and in evoked potential (EP) measures, especially in the prolonged latencies of so-called endogenous EP components, which are thought to reflect cognitive activity or information processing (Marsh and Thompson 1977; Squire et al. 1979).

As with other age-related EEG changes, the slowing of event-related potentials is far more pronounced in demented patients than in normal older adults. However, relationships between the latencies of late EP components (e.g., the P300) and performance can be shown not only in patients but also in older healthy volunteers (Pfefferbaum et al. 1982).

Age-related changes in sleep characteristics including a decrease in total sleep time and an increase in sleep latency and in the frequency of episodes of wakefulness during bedtime are accompanied by changes in the sleep EEG. During sleep there is a decrease in the proportion of time spent in the rapid eye movement (REM) and in the slow wave, i.e., deep sleep, stages 3 and 4, which are characterized by a predominance of large delta waves (Rechtschaffen and Kales 1968). Both the REM and the slow-wave sleep stages are thought to be important for the maintenance of well-being and cognitive function (Feinberg 1969).

The complementary increase in the proportion of stage 1 sleep (i.e., light sleep) and the attenuation of the regular cyclical pattern of changes in sleep stages possibly indicate a reduced capacity of the aged nervous system to maintain biological rhythms.

3.1.3   Cognitive Performance and Behavior

One of the most clearly established changes associated with normal aging is the tendency toward a decrease in the speed of behavior mediated by the CNS, including perceptual, motor, and cognitive levels of processing. This can be seen in everyday behavior as well as in the laboratory in measurements of cortical function (EEG) and in a variety of performance tasks, such as "tapping," where simple finger movements at maximum and at comfortable speed are required, in complex movements such as handwriting or tracing figures, in simple and in choice reaction time, in continuous performance tasks such as "tracking," where the movement of a target must be followed continuously (Welford 1977), in identifying targets in complex visual displays (Rabbit 1965), and in scanning tasks with memory load (e.g., "Sternberg's paradigm"; Anders and Fozard 1973).

The speed of behavioral responses tends to be disproportionally lowered in old age with more complex as compared to simple tasks, indicating a decrement mainly in the speed of central information processing (Salthouse and Somberg 1982). This can be seen, for example, in reaction time experiments with varying degrees of task complexity (Fig. 1). Limitations due to peripheral sensorimotor mechanisms should not be neglected; however, they play only a minor role in comparison to limitations imposed by central factors (Welford 1977).

Older persons tend to display increased carefulness in a wide variety of tasks, which may result in a low rate of errors at the expense of speed, when pacing of the task does not prevent this strategy (Horn and Cattell 1967). With strict pacing, forcing the subject to rapid decisions, elderly persons may respond at random due to overload, thus invalidating any measurement of response speed.

While there is a decline in the speed of central processing, which can also be seen in a number of tests of intellectual abilities involving speed, cognitive performance is not reduced in tests in which speed of response is not a crucial factor, and in particular where verbal abilities, social intelligence, and cultural knowledge are required.

These differences in the age dependency of cognitive abilities have been conceptualized as "fluid" intelligence (Cattell 1971; Horn and Cattell 1967) or "speed" performance (Oswald and Fleischmann 1985), on the one hand, and as "crystallized" intelligence or "power" performance, on the other.

Fluid intelligence is thought to represent the biological basis of cognitive functions, fundamental for the flexible processing of information, whereas crystallized intelligence largely represents acquired knowledge and thus depends on environmental factors such as education and practice.

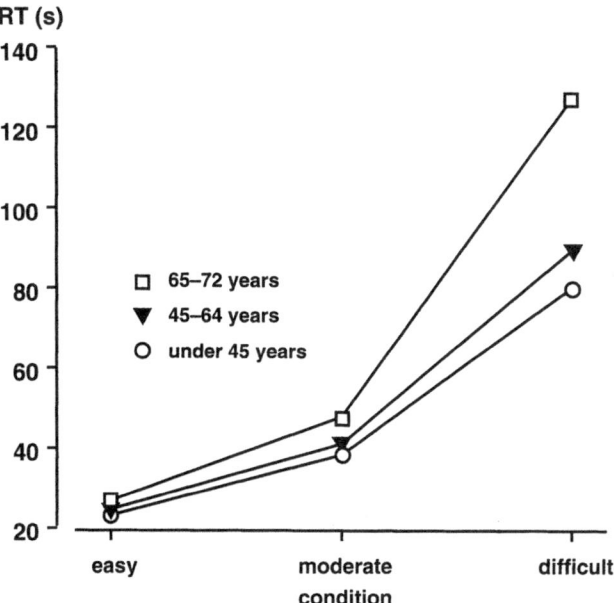

Fig. 1. Reaction times (RT) in a complex reaction time task ("spatial transposition") in healthy subjects (modified from Kay 1955)

The majority of cognition tasks used in clinical pharmacological studies aim to assess fluid components of intellectual functioning which reflect more precisely the present state of the biological system than do tests of crystallized intellectual factors.

A decline in memory performance is also a well-known phenomenon of normal aging. This is particularly true when secondary memory processes are involved, but it is not seen in primary memory (Craik 1977; Kausler 1982; Poon 1985; Wilson and Kaszniak 1986).

Primary or "working" memory is involved in the initial stage of internal processing when the material is "just in mind," at the focus of conscious attention before it is transferred to a permanent memory system (Waugh and Norman 1965).

Immediate recall of very short word lists (five to seven items) or the digit span test (Wechsler 1958) are examples of tasks in the primary memory domain, where age differences are minimal.

Secondary memory includes transferral of information to or from long-term storage, i.e., acquisition and encoding of material for storage and retrieval of stored material. In tasks involving secondary memory there are substantial age decrements. This can be seen, for example, in the recall and recognition of learned lists (words, numbers, syllables, etc.) of a length exceeding the capacity of the immediate memory span (Fig. 2).

There is some evidence that the age-related decrease is greater in free recall than in recognition, pointing to a deficit in the reconstruction of retrieval cues

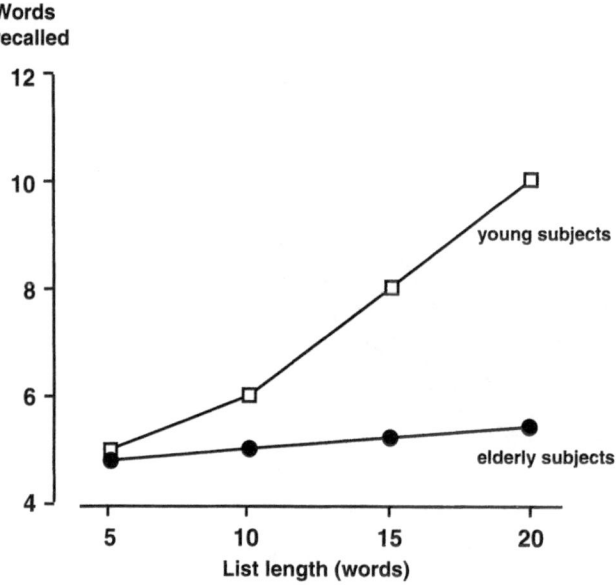

Fig. 2. Mean free recall scores (animal names) in elderly subjects aged about 70 years and young subjects aged about 20 years as a function of age and list length (modified from Craik 1968)

(Warrington and Sanders 1971). Moreover, older persons are at disproportionate disadvantage when attention cannot be fully focused on the learning material as in a "divided attention" situation (Baddeley 1986), or when the material must be reorganized for storage (Hultsch 1971). Obviously, acquisition processes are also less effective in the elderly. The decline in memory performance has been shown for verbal and nonverbal materials, in each case the age dependency being less pronounced with familiar and meaningful items than with unfamiliar or abstract materials.

Evidence for the widely held belief that only memory for recent events (as in all laboratory tasks) is affected by aging, while memory for remote events remains unimpaired, is entirely anecdotal and not supported so far by systematic research.

Age differences in learning and problem solving, where elderly persons in general perform poorer than young adults, can be attributed largely to the above-mentioned changes in the speed of information processing and in deficits in the organization and retrieval of information.

Elderly persons are handicapped particularly when the problem is unfamiliar, presents complex or conflicting information, requires switches between decision strategies, and when the solution must be found under time pressure (Rabbit 1977). They tend to adopt a risk-avoiding strategy when outcomes are predictable and may hesitate to give an affirmative response, but they may exhibit more random behavior than the young when the information load is high.

Although there is convincing evidence that cognitive factors play a major role in the age-related decrement of performance in a wide variety of laboratory tasks, the influence of motivational factors must be considered as well. Meaningfulness and perceivable relevance seem to be more important for the elderly subject's engagement in effortful coping than it is for the young. Attitude toward tests is another factor in performance. The fear of not performing well in an unfamiliar situation may actually reduce performance when defensiveness dominates behavior. The task itself may induce anxiety and concomitant reduction in performance efficiency, particularly when speed is a substantial component (Eisdorfer 1968).

It is a trivial notion that cognition and motivation, as the central factors of performance in the human information processing system, depend on both an effective sensory input and an effective motor output system.

Deficiencies in the visual and in the auditory input system are common in old age. Changes relevant to visual perception include reduced sensitivity of the eye to low quantities of light, to colors and to flicker, reduced capability for binocular depth perception, and reduced size of the visual field (Fozard et al. 1977). Deficiencies in auditory perception can be seen in a reduced threshold sensitivity for tones of high frequency ("presbycusis") or in a reduced ability for pitch discrimination and for dichotic listening.

Some of these changes cannot be explained by peripheral factors alone; deeper levels of processing are also involved, for example, in the threshold for the detection of flicker (critical flicker frequency), which is a widely accepted measure of integrative cortical function (Curran 1991; Schmidtke 1951) or in dichotic listening, which has been related to short-term memory storage (Inglis 1962).

Limitations due to effector organs producing the overt motor response include the generalized reduction in muscular strength, the reduced capacity for continued muscular effort, stiffness of joints, and reduced mobility of the neck, the latter resulting in movements of the whole body in order to see or to act sideways, where young adults perform a more parsimonious action.

Apart from the context of information processing, measures of sensory acuity and muscular capacity are useful in their own in clinical pharmacology, and the respective age-related changes must be considered carefully.

Noteworthy changes in sensory modalities, other than the visual and the auditory, include a decrease in taste sensitivity and an increase in the aversion for bitter tastes (Engen 1977), the latter possibly relevant for medication compliance; a differential decrement of vibratory sensitivity in the feet and toes relative to the fingers, most probably due to impaired circulation in the lower extremities (Goff et al. 1965); a decrease in kinesthetic capabilities, which may contribute to the more frequent occurrence of falls in old age (Kenshalo 1977); and a decrement in sensitivity to noxious stimulation associated with an increase in pain tolerance (e.g., Clark and Mehl 1971).

Pain tolerance, more than pain sensitivity, is not merely a sensory phenomenon; it is affected by motivational and cognitive factors that seem to play a greater role in older individuals' responses to pain stimulation than in young subjects' responses. Susceptibility to suggestion has been shown to influence the intensity of the experienced pain (Kenshalo 1977). Accordingly, the proportion of placebo responders reporting relief from pain after receiving a nonanalgesic substance is greater in older patients than in young (Bellville et al. 1971; Lasagna 1971; Lasagna et al. 1954).

The peripheral changes in addition to the changes in central functions must be considered in clinical pharmacology studies in order to assure the age-appropriate management and age-fair assessment of elderly individuals and hence the valid evaluation of drug effects in this population.

3.2　Cardiovascular and Pulmonary Changes

Cardiovascular and pulmonary changes in the middle-aged (defined here as 50 to 64 years) and the aged (65 years and above) population are extremely variable and very dependent upon life-style (physical activity status, smoking, malnutrition) and genetic factors (Kohn 1985; Lamy 1991; Stolarek et al. 1991; Cody 1993). The cardiovascular performance of many older subjects is no worse, or indeed better, than that of younger people, while the performance of others can be considerably below the average for their particular age group (Weisfeldt et al. 1992). Changes in cardiovascular function observed in middle-aged or aged persons may be due to clinically inapparent diseases (hypertension, coronary atherosclerosis), to life-style habits, or result simply from aging. Of these three factors, aging appears to be the least potent, and most of the changes in cardiovascular function that are induced solely be aging are clinically important only when they are superimposed on significant diseases or cardiovascular or pulmonary stresses (Weisfeldt et al. 1992).

3.2.1　Heart

Cardiopulmonary changes can be observed between the ages of 50 and 60 years using appropriate methods (Weisfeldt et al. 1992). Under resting conditions, however, they often remain clinically insignificant, unless the cardiovascular and pulmonary systems are compromised, especially by toxic environmental substances or nicotine abuse. After the age of 60 to 65 years, however, more marked physical changes occur (Lindenfeld and Groves 1982; Cody 1993). Under normal circumstances the aging heart can indeed adapt, and an average level of activity can be maintained (Brandfonbrener et al. 1955). Anatomic changes (loss of muscle fibers, moderate hypertrophy of left ventricular myocardium, increased amount of collagenous material), and physiological alterations (alterations of the conduction system, loss of contractile efficiency, decrease in cardiac β-adrenoreceptor responsiveness) lead to diminished contractility and filling capacity (Port et al. 1980; Proper and Wall 1972; Gerstenblith et al. 1977) and cause reduced stroke volume and diminished cardiac output at rest (when measured with invasive methodology, whereas noninvasive methods show no significant age-related decreases in cardiac output, stroke volume, or ejection fraction).

The ability of the myocardium to generate tension is often well maintained as a result of prolonged duration of contraction and greater stiffness, despite a modest decrease in the velocity of shortening of cardiac muscle. An increased stiffness and delayed relaxation may limit the early left ventricular filling during stress, although end-diastolic volume is not compromised in healthy persons.

More relevant changes are found during exercise stress (Myers and Froelicher 1990). The increase in heart rate as the typical response to stress becomes less effective (Yin et al. 1978; Port et al. 1980; Rodeheffer et al. 1984), even in the very fit (Hagberg et al. 1985). The heart begins to have difficulty adapting to its workload (Table 1), especially when unusual demands are made on it. Furthermore, the heart rate required to maintain optimal circulatory function narrows in range and even mild tachycardia or bradycardia may lead to a relevant deficit in blood flow in vital organs.

Table 1. Effect of age on cardiac index and heart rate at rest and during exercise (modified from Kennedy and Caird 1981)

	Age range (years)			
	30	50	60	70
Resting heart rate (bpm)	76	68	66	62
Maximum heart rate (bpm)	182	174	164	155
Cardiac index ($l\ min^{-1}\ m^{-2}$)	3.5	2.8–3.1	2.6–3.7	2.4–3.6

The influence of aging on maximum oxygen consumption (Dehn and Bruce 1971), the best index of cardiovascular performance, is unclear due to difficulties in determining this particular parameter in aged persons. This is because musculoskeletal problems often restrict the workload before the true maximum oxygen consumption is achieved, and age differences in muscle mass can furthermore bias the test results.

3.2.2 Blood Pressure

Arterial blood vessels are affected more than the heart by changes in aging as they undergo progressive stiffness due to a loss of elastin and smooth muscles and due to an increased amount of collagen, which together with the development of an atherosclerosis leads to increased peripheral resistance (Lakatta 1989; Morgenstern and Byyny 1992). These arterial changes are widespread and result in diminished circulation to all organs and tissues, of which the effects on brain perfusion and kidney circulation (reduction in renal plasma flow) and the effects on peripheral blood pressure are the most relevant: the systolic arterial blood pressure gradually increases with age due to the decreased aortic elasticity (and is in part responsible for the mild left ventricular hypertrophy), whereas the less marked increase in diastolic blood pressure results from the increased resistance in the peripheral arterial blood vessels (Byyny 1990; Klein et al. 1990; Michelsen and Otterstad 1990).

The blood pressure response during maximum exercise is greater in subjects aged over 50 years than in younger counterparts, whereas the heart rate during exercise is lower in older than in younger subjects (Michelsen and Otterstad 1990; Table 2).

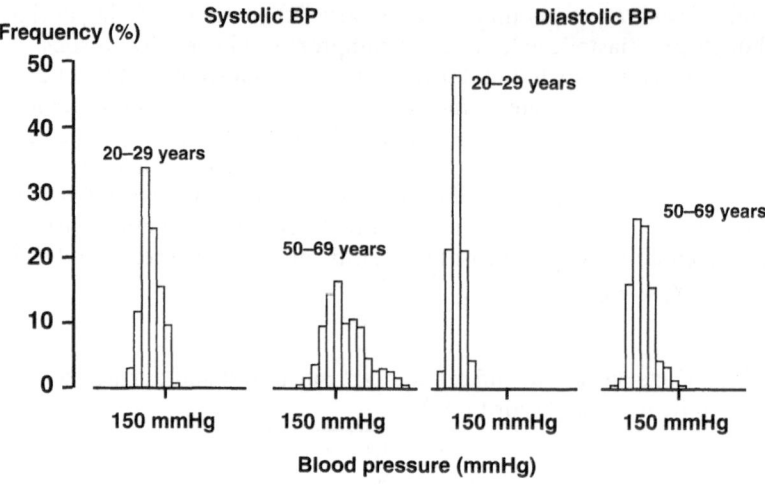

Fig. 3. Frequency distribution of systolic and diastolic blood pressure in 244 women aged 10–29 years and 97 women aged 50–69 years (redrawn from Pickering 1968). In the older group the peak of frequency drifts towards higher blood pressure values, and the distribution becomes broader (150 mmHg is marked as a reference, the scale of the abscissa is identical)

Another relevant finding is the broad frequency distribution of both systolic and diastolic blood pressure (Fig. 3) in the elderly compared with young subjects (Pickering 1968).

The increases in blood pressure with age are also demonstrable with 24-h blood pressure monitoring (Table 3) but are less marked (Cox et al. 1991; O'Brien et al. 1991; Kennedy et al. 1983).

Table 2. Changes in systolic and diastolic blood pressure (mmHg) with age

		Age range (years)				
	Sex	30–39	40–49	50–59	60–69	50–79
Systolic BP at rest[a]	Men	125 ± 9	129 ± 10	133 ± 15	135 ± 14	—
	Women	117 ± 11	119 ± 10	120 ± 14	136 ± 18	—
Systolic BP at rest[b]	Men	122 ± 11	125 ± 16	—	—	133 ± 15
	Women	113 ± 10	121 ± 17	—	—	130 ± 24
Diastolic BP at rest[a]	Men	76 ± 6	74 ± 9	82±7	83± 6	—
	Women	73 ± 6	75 ± 5	74 ± 9	80 ± 9	—
Diastolic BP at rest[b]	Men	77 ± 8	81 ± 10	—	—	85 ± 11
	Women	72 ± 8	78 ± 9	—	—	81 ± 12
Systolic BP during maximal exercise[a]	Men	182 ± 27	192 ± 21	197 ± 21	206 ± 23	—
	Women	163 ± 16	168 ± 19	171 ± 26	190 ± 20	—
Diastolic BP during maximal exercise[a]	Men	76 ± 6	74 ± 9	82 ± 7	83 ± 6	—
	Women	73 ± 6	75 ± 5	74 ± 9	80 ± 9	—

[a] From Michelsen and Otterstadt 1990.

[b] From O'Brien et al. 1990.

Table 3. Ambulatory 24-h blood pressure (mmHg) monitoring: changes in mean systolic and diastolic blood pressure during daytime period with age

		Age range (years)				
		30–39	40–49	50–79	17–49	50–80
Daytime systolic BP[a]	Men	128 ± 9	129 ± 12	132 ± 12		
	Women	117 ± 8	121 ± 12	126 ± 18		
Daytime diastolic BP[a]	Men	80 ± 6	83 ± 9	84 ± 9		
	Women	75 ± 7	76 ± 9	78 ± 9		
Daytime systolic BP[b]	Men				129 ± 9	132 ± 12
	Women				118 ± 7	129 ± 15
Daytime diastolic BP[b]	Men				81 ± 9	85 ± 9
	Women				75 ± 6	79 ± 8

[a] From O'Brien et al. 1991.

[b] From Cox et al. 1991.

Baroreceptor function, which plays a major role in blood pressure regulation via tonic regulation of the activity of the vasomotor center, is diminished in the elderly (Gribbin et al. 1971). As a consequence, elderly persons are more prone to experience a decrease in blood pressure when baroreceptor function is required to maintain circulatory homeostasis, such as when standing up or after tilting (Vargas et al. 1986; Vita et al. 1986; Hainsworth and Al-Shamma 1988; Piha 1991). Hypotensive blood pressure responses to posture change and postprandial blood pressure reductions are commonly observed in many old subjects (Lipsitz 1989) and vary greatly from day to day.

3.2.3 Arrhythmias

Arrhythmias (tachyarrhythmias and bradyarrhythmias) occur more frequently in the elderly than in young adolescents. This may be due in part to the increasing prevalence of hypertension and coronary artery disease but also applies to elderly persons without any incidence of organic heart disease (Manayari et al. 1990; Bethge et al. 1983; Bjerregaard 1982; Kennedy et al. 1977, 1981; Fleg and Kennedy 1982; Manz et al. 1990).

3.2.4 Lung

The respiratory system is subject to quite relevant changes with aging that are often not obvious at rest but nearly always demonstrable during exercise. A progressive loss of elasticity and changes in the structure of the chest can lead to difficulties in expiration (Martin et al. 1979; Thurlbeck and Angus 1975). Total lung capacity is mostly unchanged, but vital capacity is gradually and progressively reduced (Fig. 4). The forced expiratory volume and the maximum breathing capacity are both diminished, while the residual volume and the expiratory reserve volume are increased. The partial pressure of arterial oxygen (PaO_2) declines with age, but in healthy elderly persons the partial pressure

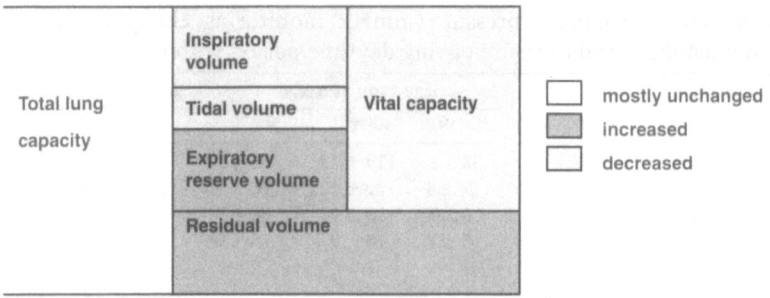

Fig. 4. Changes in lung volume with aging (modified from McDaniel 1992)

of carbon dioxide (PCO2) remains unaffected. These functional deficits generally do not impair pulmonary function of healthy elderly subjects at rest or during
minimal exercise, but even after only moderate stress elderly persons are at risk
of respiratory failure (diminished PaO2, increased PCO2, drop in arterial pH),
and these deficits are an important reason for the increased susceptibility of the
elderly to pulmonary and bronchial infections (Culver and Butler 1985).

The normal alterations in pulmonary function with aging are furthermore often superimposed by pulmonary changes due to chronic environmental
pollution (smoking, pollution by various industrial agents), which cause
decreased ciliary action and increased mucus production. These pollutants
increase the age-related obstructive components, have per se a negative effect
on pulmonary and cardiovascular function, and thus aggravate the age-related
changes in pulmonary function. The potential of unrecognized changes in
pulmonary function is present in all persons over the age of 40 to 50 years.

3.3   Changes in Clinical Chemistry and Hematology

Traditionally, clinical chemical and hematological variables are studied to detect
functional or metabolic disorders and toxic or allergic disturbances. Results outside predetermined reference limits suggest alterations of body function and the
need for further investigations.

However, interpreting laboratory test results in older subjects can be difficult
as the aging process can shift hematological and clinical chemistry parameters
outside the "normal" range of conventional population-based reference values,
which are generally established from younger subjects. A correct interpretation
of laboratory test results in the elderly is furthermore complicated by the fact
that, even if reference ranges for the elderly exist, they are biased inasmuch as
inapparent diseases or even known codiseases and comedications are often not
considered. Yet these are frequently present in the elderly population and can
alter hematological and clinical chemistry test results considerably. Even in
reports of hematological and biochemical ranges established from "true" healthy
elderly subjects, study results are necessarily influenced by diseases that are not
clinically manifest.

In addition, several clinical chemistry and hematological parameters are subject to significant individual variability with regard to the "personal" normal value in an individual person (Table 4). These parameters demonstrate a higher within-subject than between-subject variation, thereby rendering reference ranges practically useless. In these cases, screening using the conventional reference limits is unlikely to detect early disorders because many persons have values outside their individual reference limits while classified as "normal." Only repeated measurements from individual subjects permit an analysis of whether a critical range has been exceeded, or whether a nonrandom trend has occurred (Fraser 1989).

Table 4. Indices of variability in some clinical chemistry and hematological parameters (within-subject variation/between subject variation) in the elderly (from Fraser 1989)

Creatinine	0.23
Alkaline phosphatase	0.27
Calcium	0.58
Potassium	0.71
Albumin	0.74
Urea	0.77
Sodium	0.98
Mean cell hemoglobin	0.21
Mean cell volume	0.27
Erythrocyte count	0.32
Platelet count	0.40
Hemoglobin	0.43
Hematocrit	0.44
Leukocyte count	0.58

Values >1.4 indicate reference values satisfactory for monitoring changes while values < 0.6 are of little use.

A relevant aspect in the evaluation of clinical chemistry and hematological parameters in the elderly is that even when the means of the variables are not relevantly different from those of young subjects, the reference ranges can be broader in the former (Jernigan et al. 1980; Thompson 1988).

Within-subject variations of clinical chemistry (Table 5) and hematological parameters in the elderly are probably similar to those of young persons (Fraser et al. 1989b; Fraser 1993), indicating that this aspect of homeostasis might not be compromised in the elderly. However, this is still a matter of controversy.

3.3.1 Clinical Chemistry

Several authors have published clinical chemistry data from elderly persons, often in relatively small samples sizes and in populations which are not necessarily representative of elderly subjects in clinical trials. The most comprehensive data on young and elderly persons has recently been published

Table 5. Mean within-subject variation (%) in clinical chemistry parameters in young and elderly subjects (modified from Fraser 1993)

	Young	Elderly
Alkaline phosphatase	9.8	6.5
Total bilirubin	19.2	16.5
Creatinine	4.1	4.3
Urea	13.9	10.3
Total protein	3.1	2.6
Albumin	2.2	2.6
Total cholesterol	5.8	4.9
Triglycerides	17.5	15.3
Glucose	4.8	4.7
Sodium	0.7	0.9
Potassium	5.4	4.8
Chloride	1.2	1.2
Calcium	2.1	1.6

by Tietz et al. (1992), but even in this impressive analysis the investigated elderly subjects were not really healthy. However, the numerous data on laboratory findings in the elderly population provide a basis for evaluating trends and a global overview of changes with age.

Blood urea nitrogen (BUN), alkaline phosphatase, and creatinine in serum increase progressively with age, in men more so than in women (Kelly et al. 1979; Leask et al. 1973; Hale et al. 1983; Tietz et al. 1984; Dybkaer et al. 1981), which might be explained by age-related parenchymal changes that affect both glomerular filtration and tubular functions. Total plasma protein and total plasma albumin, on the other hand, decline with age (Leask et al. 1973; Campion et al. 1988; Greenblatt et al. 1979).

Serum bilirubin remains within the range of young subjects or decreases slightly with age (Hale et al. 1983); serum cholesterol and triglycerides are undoubtedly affected both by age and sex, with wide reference ranges, and decreases slightly after the age of 75 (Leask et al. 1973).

Lactic dehydrogenase (LDH) increases with age, more so in women than in men. SGOT, SGPT, glucose, and uric acid do not differ from values measured in young subjects (Hale et al. 1983; West and Ash 1984). The normal range of glycosylated hemoglobin (HbA1) in elderly subjects does not differ from established reference ranges in younger patients (Mulkerrin et al. 1992).

Serum electrolytes (sodium, potassium, chloride, and bicarbonate) in the healthy elderly are generally within the normal range of young subjects (Hale et al. 1983); only calcium declines with age (Leask et al. 1973), whereas electrolyte imbalance is common in geriatric patients (Adams and Martin 1991).

Beginning at puberty mean plasma renin activity and plasma renin levels decline in healthy subjects, with wide variations in individual values, and reach their lowest levels during the sixth decade of life (Bauer 1993). Similarly, plasma aldosterone levels and urinary excretion of aldosterone decrease gradually. The mechanisms for the age-related decrease in plasma renin activity are unknown and considered to be the primary cause of low aldosterone values in older adults. These changes in elderly subjects are generally only modest and do not alter fluid or electrolyte metabolism but can precipitate the development of hyperkalemia in elderly subjects.

Plasma osmolality, as an objective assessment of hydration, is not influenced by age (Woo and Swaminathan 1991). Higher values of mean plasma osmolality found in previous studies of unselected elderly subjects might reflect the higher incidence of diseases in the elderly.

Table 6 summarizes the changes in clinical chemistry parameters with age as relative ratios of median values.

Table 6. Changes in clinical chemistry parameters with age (men aged 30 years taken as 1.00; modified from Fraser 1993)

	Sex	Age (years)			
		30	50	65	80
Alkaline phosphatase	Men	1.00	1.07	1.15	1.15
	Women	0.82	0.90	0.95	0.95
AST (SGOT)	Men	1.00	1.01	1.02	1.03
	Women	0.82	0.90	0.95	0.95
ALT (SGPT)	Men	1.00	1.05	0.91	0.80
	Women	0.64	0.75	0.75	0.69
LDH	Men	1.00	1.03	1.03	1.07
	Women	0.93	1.02	1.08	1.10
Total bilirubin	Men	1.00	0.95	0.95	1.02
	Women	0.80	0.80	0.75	0.75
Creatinine	Men	1.00	1.02	1.03	1.05
	Women	0.83	0.85	0.85	0.85
Urea	Men	1.00	1.04	1.10	1.20
	Women	0.85	0.95	1.05	1.10
Total protein	Men	1.00	0.99	0.98	0.96
	Women	0.98	0.98	0.97	0.96
Albumin	Men	1.00	0.96	0.93	0.88
	Women	0.97	0.95	0.92	0.88
Total cholesterol	Men	1.00	1.12	1.12	1.05
	Women	0.98	1.13	1.18	1.15
Triglycerides	Men	1.00	1.15	1.10	<1.05
	Women	0.75	0.90	1.05	>1.20
Sodium	Men	1.00	1.00	1.00	1.00
	Women	1.00	1.00	1.00	1.00
Potassium	Men	1.00	1.02	1.03	1.05
	Women	0.99	1.00	1.02	1.00
Chloride	Men	1.00	1.00	1.00	1.00
	Women	1.00	1.00	1.00	1.00
Calcium	Men	1.00	0.98	0.97	0.96
	Women	0.97	0.98	0.97	0.98

3.3.2 Hematology

Leukocyte counts in the elderly do not differ from those of young subjects (Hale et al. 1983; Mattila et al. 1986) or are reported to be lower (Tietz et al. 1992; Zauber and Zauber 1987), whereas the presence of age-related changes in erythrocytes is unclear (Zauber and Zauber 1987; Besa 1988; Zaino 1981; Corberand et al. 1987). Hemoglobin and hematocrit decline with age, and the rate of decline is greater in men than in women. The erythrocyte sedimentation rate tends to increase with age, particularly in women (Hanger et al. 1991a). However, changes in the elderly may be caused by variations of other variables such as hemoglobin, albumin or fibrinogen, possibly as a result of disease states, rather than age per se. The elderly have lower vitamin B12 levels but higher red cell and serum folate levels (Marcus et al. 1987; Hangar et al. 1991b). Table 7 summarizes changes in hematological variables with age.

Table 7. Changes in hematological parameters with age in mixed population (in part with codiseases and comedication; summary from several publications)

	Increased	Decreased	Same as young subjects
Leukocytes	–	–	+
Erythrocytes	–	?	?
Hemoglobin, Hematocrit	–	+	–
ESR	+	–	–
Vitamin B12	–	+	–
Red cell and serum folate	+	–	–

3.3.3   Repeated Measurements of Clinical Chemistry and Hematological Variables

While the clinician performs repeated measurements to demonstrate that a pathological variable has returned to normal, the clinical pharmacologist seeks primarily to demonstrate that a particular variable remains constant over time, which is methodologically more elaborate and assumes some knowledge of the "normal" course of the variable.

The calculation of the "critical difference" (Dcrit) is a very appropriate method for this. Although a very simple method that provides valid criteria for interpreting the results of repeated measurements (Lienert 1969), it has unfortunately not found a wide audience in either clinical practice or in scientific, and in particular clinical pharmacological research. The critical difference describes the changes in a variable (as an absolute value or as a percentage change) which lie within the normal range of scatter during follow-up investigations, i.e., two or more repeated measurements. Values above the critical difference are statistically significant, without necessarily indicating a pathological change. For instance, a Dcrit of 10 U/l for SGPT (ALT) would mean that, with a baseline value of 16 U/l, a follow-up value of 25 U/l would still lie within the expected range of variability and thus be insignificant, although an isolated value of 25 U/l lies outside the reference range.

Various approaches to calculating critical difference have been put forward in the literature (Lienert 1969; Costongs et al. 1984; Fraser and Fogarty 1989; Queraltó et al. 1993), but in the main they all arrive at comparable results and are based on a consideration of methodological and biological variances and the correlation between repeated measurements. The approach of Lienert has proven particularly practicable and has for many years been applied in experimental psychology. Table 8 presents an overview of the critical differences of clinical chemistry variables in healthy subjects, as described by the various authors. Table 9 shows the relationship between the observation period and the size of the critical difference.

Table 8. Critical differences (in absolute units) in clinical chemistry test results in serial tests (from Costongs et al. 1984; Fraser and Fogarty 1989; Queraltó et al. 1993)

Alkaline phosphatase (U/l)	11–26
LDH (U/l)	41–181
SGPT (ALT) (U/l)	9–33
SGOT (AST) (U/l)	6–18
γ-GT (U/l)	15–33
Total bilirubin (μmol/l)	4–6
Creatinine (μmol/l)	14 -25
Urea (μmol/l)	1.6–3.2
Total protein (g/l)	5–8.7
Albumin (g/)	4–6.8
Total cholesterol (mmol/l)	0.9 -1.9
Triglycerides (mmol/l)	0.6–1.8
Glucose, fasting (mmol/l)	0.9–1.9
Sodium (mmol/l)	4.0–8.8
Potassium (mmol/l)	0.5–0.85
Chloride (mmol/l)	5–9
Calcium (mmol/l)	0.12–0.37

Table 9. Critical differences in clinical chemistry variables after short-term and long-term observations (from Costongs et al. 1985a–c)

	After 1 day	After 6 months
Alkaline phosphatase	14.6	41.3
LDH	28.1	50.4
SGPT (ALT)	29.2	134.4
SGOT (AST)	26.7	71.6
γ-GT	36.4	74.2
Total bilirubin	70.6	81.0
Creatinine	19.8	38.7
Urea	27.9	53.7
Total protein	13.8	14.9
Albumin	15.0	18.3
Total cholesterol	18.8	35.2
Triglycerides	96.2	97.1
Glucose, fasting	73.1	59.0
Sodium	4.3	4.0
Potassium	22.2	20.8
Chloride	7.4	7.4
Calcium	10.4	12.1
Calcium thromboplastin time	7.8	34.2
Activated partial thromboplastin time	29.0	37.2
Thrombin time	18.1	21.7
Fibrinogen	37.8	54.2

There have been no specific studies of critical differences in elderly subjects participating in clinical pharmacological trials.

3.3.4 Biological Rhythms

Circannual rhythms (Nicolau and Haus 1989) have been described in several laboratory parameters of elderly subjects, but the majority of them have no relevant implications for the interpretation of test results, whereas daily (cortisol), monthly (follicle-stimulating hormone, luteinizing hormone), or seasonal (cholesterol) rhythms in some quantities are of significant importance.

3.4 Changes in Pharmacokinetics

In the main, changes in pharmacokinetics with increasing age are secondary consequences of an alteration of one or more body systems or are due to general aging processes that influence the kinetic factors distribution and excretion. They are hardly ever due to real changes in basic intracellular metabolism. Table 10 summarizes the changes in body function and their impact on drug disposition.

3.4.1 Absorption

Although age-dependent changes in various physiological parameters suggest some alteration in drug absorption, no such finding has ever been demonstrated. Gastric emptying rate, gastrointestinal motility, and gastrointestinal blood flow decrease with age while gastric pH increases, but only few and clinically insignificant changes in the rate or extent of drug absorption have been observed in the elderly population, as most drugs are absorbed by passive diffusion, and thus the normal aging process has only a minor impact on drug absorption.

3.4.2 Distribution

No direct relationship has been demonstrated between the volume of distribution and age. However, total body weight declines steadily after the age of 50–60 years, primarily due to a 10%–15% loss of intracellular water (Novak 1972; Hollister 1981), and lean body mass decreases (Barlett et al. 1991), while there is a relative increase in fat tissue mass of 20%–50%. Thus the volume of distribution of many drugs must be expected to be different in young and elderly subjects, and alterations in body fat with aging may lead to an accumulation of drugs that are highly lipid soluble (Tsujimoto et al. 1989a).

Furthermore, alterations in regional blood flow or changes in the integrity of the blood-brain barrier may affect the distribution of drugs, but systematic studies have yet to confirm this assumption.

Table 10. Effect of alterations in body functions with age on pharmacokinetic processes (modified from Vestal 1978)

Kinetic process	Physiological function	Alteration in elderly	Influence on kinetics
Absorption			
	Gastric acid secretion	↓	
	Gastric pH	↑	
	Blood flow in gut	↓	→ Not demonstrable
	Number of gastric cells	↓	
	Gastrointestinal motility	↓	
Distribution			
	Total body water	↓	→ Influence on Vd and
	Lean body weight	↓	plasma concentration
	Body fat	↑	LD: Vd, delayed excretion
	Protein binding		
	Serum albumin	↓	
	α-Glycoprotein	↑ or ↔	→ Changes in unbound
	γ-Globulin	↑ or ↔	fraction
	RBC binding	↓ or ↔	
Metabolism			
	Hepatic blood flow	↓	→ Decreased hepatic
	Hepatic mass	↓	clearance
Excretion			
	Renal plasma flow	↓	
	Number of nephrons	↓	→ RD: decreased renal
	Glomerular filtration rate	↓	clearance, prolonged $t^{1}/_{2}$
	Tubular secretion	↓	

LD, Lipophile drugs; RD, drugs with relevant renal excretion; Vd, volume of distribution.

3.4.3 Protein Binding

Protein binding is an important determinant of the rate of metabolism of drugs that are capacity limited.

The concentration of serum albumin may be decreased in the elderly (Veering et al. 1990), thus leading to an increase in the unbound fraction of highly protein bound (i.e., more than 90% of total plasma drug) substances, whereas the basic binding affinity of albumin to drug is not reduced with age (Triggs and Nation 1975). However, rate and amount of glomerular filtration of drugs is dependent on the degree of protein binding, thus minimizing an increase in unbound drug. In general, changes in protein binding can independently affect both the drug distribution and the clearance (which as independent parameters both determine the half-life of a drug in the body).

Concentration of γ-globulin and α-glycoprotein in elderly subjects is unchanged (Veering et al. 1990); drug binding to erythrocytes might be lower.

3.4.4 Metabolism

Drug metabolism takes place primarily in the liver, but to a limited extent also in other organs such as the kidney and the lungs. Age-related histological changes in the liver are minor and of uncertain significance; many standard function tests do not change significantly with aging, but hepatic drug metabolism is often significantly influenced by aging processes.

Intracellular hepatic function, i.e., the activity of the hepatic microsomal drug-metabolizing enzyme systems, does not seem — in contrast to studies in rodents (Kato and Takanaka 1968; McMartin et al. 1980) — to be influenced in healthy humans by age (Woodhouse and Wynne 1988, 1992; Wynne et al. 1989; Williams et al. 1989a; Schmucker et al. 1990; Herd et al. 1991; Hunt et al. 1992). There is, however, some evidence of a selective impairment in the activity of some cytochrome P450 isoenzymes in the healthy elderly population (Posner et al. 1987; Chandler et al. 1988). In general, phase I reactions (mainly oxidation, catalyzed by the cytochrome P450 system on the smooth endoplasmic reticulum of hepatocytes) seem to be more age-dependent than phase II biotransformations, i.e., synthetic or conjugation steps in the cytosol or plasma (Greenblatt et al. 1982b). Age-related decreases in the clearance due to reduced hepatic oxidation have been described for example for high-clearance drugs such as clormethiazole (Nation et al. 1977), nicardipine (Forette et al. 1989) and nifedipine (Robertson et al. 1988) and due to reduced conjugation for lorazepam (Greenblatt et al. 1979) and paracetamol (Wynne et al. 1990a). The data available suggest furthermore that many of these changes seen in the elderly are more pronounced and more relevant in disease states and in frailty (Williams et al. 1989b).

More important for drug disposure are age-related decreases in hepatic blood flow and hepatic volume, which explain the reduced hepatic clearance of many drugs in the elderly (Bach et al. 1981; Swift et al. 1978):

- Hepatic blood flow decreases with age by up to 35% (Wynne et al. 1989), which necessarily reduces the rate of drug metabolism of highly flow-dependent substances such as propranolol and others (Table 11).
- Hepatic weight (Calloway et al. 1965) and volume (Swift et al. 1978) are reduced in the elderly (about 25%). This decline in functional hepatic mass is probably the most important alteration with regard to pharmacokinetics that occurs in the human liver with aging (Marchesini et al. 1990).

Table 11. Changes in clearance, volume of distribution (Vd), and terminal half life ($t_{1/2}$) of some flow-dependent, highly extracted drugs with age (modified from Tsujimoto et al. 1989)

Drug	Age	Vd (l/kg)	$t_{1/2}$ (h)	Cl (ml/min/kg)
Indocyanine green	Young	41.6 ± 6.4	3.1 ± 0.3 min	7.1 ± 1.2
	Elderly	41.1 ± 5.3	4.7 ± 0.6 min	6.1 ± 0.6
Propranolol	Young	3.8 ± 0.3	4.5 ± 0.4 h	10.6 ± 1.3
	Elderly	4.2 ± 0.5	5.6 ± 0.6 h	9.0 ± 0.9
Morphine	Young	3.2 ± 0.3	3.0 ± 0.5 h	14.7 ± 0.9
	Elderly	4.7 ± 0.2	4.4 ± 0.3 h	12.4 ± 1.2

Presystemic and first-pass metabolism, which reduce bioavailability of a drug, decline in some drugs significantly with age, for example, propranolol (Castleden and George 1979) or labetalol (Kelly et al. 1982).

Induction responses of some enzymes in human liver may be reduced with aging (Vestal et al. 1979b); however, this blunting of enzyme induction responses in old age may be due merely to the reduced use of common inducers such as cigarettes and alcohol.

3.4.5 Excretion

Drugs or their metabolites are excreted mainly via bile or urine. Data on the effect of age on biliary excretion of drugs are scant; animal data give some indication of an impairment of hepatobiliary function with age. Relevant effects of age on drug excretion have only been described for the kidney, which is for some drugs and/or their metabolites the exclusive route of elimination (by glomerular filtration, tubular secretion and tubular reabsorption).

Renal plasma flow (estimated by PAH clearance) and glomerular filtration rate (GFR), as measured by inulin clearance or endogenous creatinine clearance, decrease with age (Rowe et al. 1976; Davies and Shock 1950). The creatinine serum concentration, however, rises only insignificantly or even decreases, since creatinine production from the muscles decreases mostly at the same rate as the renal clearance of creatinine, which is caused by a decrease in body muscle mass in the elderly (Table 12). Determination of single point serum creatinine concentrations for modifying dosages of renally excreted drugs can therefore be misleading.

Table 12. Changes in creatinine clearance, creatinine excretion, and creatinine serum concentrations with age (modified from Rowe et al. 1976)

Age (years)	Creatinine clearance (ml/min/1.73 m^2)	Serum creatinine (mg/dl)	Creatinine excretion (mg/24 h)
25–34	140.1	0.81	1862
35–44	132.6	0.81	1746
45–54	126.8	0.83	1689
55–64	119.9	0.84	1580
65–74	109.5	0.83	1409
75–84	96.9	0.84	1259

The reduction in GFR is necessarily bound to a reduced renal excretion of all drugs that are eliminated mainly by the kidneys. This alteration of renal excretion rate is the most important pharmacokinetic change in the older population, but it must be stressed that a decline in renal function is not an inevitable consequence of aging (Lindeman et al. 1985; Lindeman 1992), since one-third of elderly persons have no decrease in renal function.

Other renal processes that influence the excretion of drugs are active tubular reabsorption, tubular secretion, and nonionic back diffusion (passive reabsorption), which are important pathways for highly protein-bound substances. Renal tubular cells appear to exhibit a protein uncoupling mechanism as protein-bound drugs are not filtered but readily secreted from blood to tubular lumen. These processes may be altered in the elderly simply by a loss in the number of nephrons (without basic defect of the individual tubules); another negative impact on tubular secretion of drugs is the development of dehydration accompanying a frequent loss of thirst, even in healthy older subjects (Philips et al. 1984). The resultant reduction in tubular reabsorption, i.e., due to an inability to concentrate sodium and water, increases the urinary loss of drugs such as lithium. From the practical point of view, however, it is important that these tubular functions closely parallel the decreases in GFR with age. Therefore, the measurement of creatinine clearance provides all the information necessary to estimate drug clearance for substances that are cleared totally or partially unchanged by the kidneys (Lindeman 1992).

Taking together all data on changes in drug disposition in healthy elderly subjects, it must be concluded that not all, but many drugs undergo changes in their pharmacokinetic behavior, which may lead to significantly increased plasma concentrations and relevantly delayed drug excretion. Since these changes are to a large extent unpredictable in the majority of drugs and of individual subjects, it is reasonable to start treatment with smaller doses of a drug in elderly healthy subjects (and even more in elderly with diseases) than in younger subjects, for instance, with two-thirds of a young adult maintenance dose. However, it is difficult to make general rules about kinetic changes in the elderly, and each drug must be tested separately.

3.5   Changes in Receptor Sensitivity

Clinical experience has shown that the elderly differ from younger adults in their sensitivity to a number of different drugs. Explanations of these changes in drug responsiveness have focused mainly on assessing modifications of pharmacokinetics in the former. Age-related kinetic changes can result in a different drug availability, with consequent alterations in pharmacodynamic effects. Differences in drug effectiveness between the different age groups need not, however, simply be the result of pharmacokinetic changes alone. Rather, modifications at the receptor sites where drugs are bound and start the reactions which finally result in the pharmacological action can produce different pharmacodynamic effects in elderly persons which are not related to altered kinetics (Crooks 1983). The investigation of this aspect, however, is much more difficult than that of pharmacokinetic changes.

In general, a change in drug response is reflected by a shift in the drug's dose-response curve (Wood and Feely 1985). This can occur as a result of a change in the total number of receptors at the various target tissues or can be due to change in the "sensitivity" of the receptors. The relation between drug, receptor and pharmacological effect is generally described by the formula

$$[D] + [R] \overset{K_1}{\underset{K_2}{\leftrightarrow}} [DR] \rightarrow E$$

where: $[D]$ = free drug concentration at the receptor site, $[R]$ = number of receptors not occupied by the drug, $[DR]$ = drug-receptor complex which depends on the binding constant k_1 and the dissociation constant k_2, and $[E]$ = resultant effect.

According to this formula, a strict delineation of pharmacokinetics and pharmacodynamics is only arbitrary, because both are inseparable factors when considering the clinical effects of a drug (Shillingford and Shillingford 1987).

Many studies of age-related changes in receptor sensitivity have dealt with the autonomic nervous system. Summarizing the findings, there is considerable evidence that the β-adrenergic responsiveness to a number of different physiological and pharmacological stimuli is decreased in elderly subjects (Palmer at el. 1978; Saar and Gordon 1979; Rowe and Troen 1980). This may be due to a reduction in the number of β-receptors and/or the drug affinity to the different binding sites (Schocken and Roth 1977), or due to changes in the postreceptor reactions, for example, declines in adenylate cyclase and cAMP phosphodiesterase activities, which are finally responsible for the clinical effect (Lakatta and Yin 1982; Roth and Hess 1982; Feldman et al. 1983, 1984).

Many studies have demonstrated that the effectiveness of β-receptor agonists decreases with the age of the patient, resulting in a reduced β1- and β2-adrenergic modulation of the cardiovascular system (Guarnieri et al. 1980; van Brummelen et al. 1981; Rodeheffer et al. 1984; Fleg et al. 1985; Docherty 1986; Scarpace et al. 1991). It is not clear, however, whether this desensitization is due to an age-related reduction in receptor binding. Interaction studies with different antagonists that bind specifically to β-receptor sites have produced contradictory findings: the decreased receptor sensitivity to propanolol suggests an age-related change in receptor binding, whereas timolol indicates no reduction in the elderly (Vestal et al. 1979a; Klein et al. 1986).

Summarizing the findings, the most widely proposed conception of age-related β-adrenoceptor changes are a functional defect in the postreceptor reactions (Feldman et al. 1984) and a reduction in the high affinity binding sites of β-receptors (Docherty 1986; O'Malley et al. 1987).

The effects of the stimulation of cholinergic receptors on the cardiovascular system are distinctly diminished with increasing age. A less pronounced reduction in heart rate occurs in older people after vagal stimulation than in young adults. On the other hand, atropine clearly enhances heart rate to a lesser extent in the elderly than in the young (Kelliher and Conahan 1980). Likewise, the effects of most anticholinergic drugs are decreased, while the untoward effects are more severe in aged subjects. The basic principles of these changes, however, are still unknown.

Thus, the combined changes in the β-adrenergic and the cholinergic receptor actions, i.e., of the autonomic sympathetic and parasympathetic nervous control of the cardiovascular system, may explain the complex physiological modifications in heart and vascular functions with advancing age per se and after treatment with drugs which act on one or both systems.

In contrast to the β-adrenergic and the cholinergic receptor systems, α-adrenergic reactions appear not to undergo any clinically relevant change with age (Kendall et al. 1982; Scott et al. 1988).

More firm conclusions are permitted about the decreased baroreceptor sensitivity in the elderly. The well-known increase in arterial wall stiffness prevents an adequate reaction of these mechanoreceptors to blood pressure changes. Moreover, the impaired function of this system may account — via reduced inhibition of the central nervous vasomotor center — for the increased basal blood pressure and the enhanced responses to hemodynamic stimulations in the elderly (Kohn 1977).

From epidemiological studies, for example, the Boston Collaboratory Drug Surveillance Program (Greenblatt 1977), it is known that the elderly exhibit a greater responsiveness to various central acting drugs, in particular after chronic medication. An exaggeration of the pharmacological effects in elderly patients, especially the increased incidence of severe adverse events, may result from an increased sensitivity of the benzodiazepine receptors. Diazepam, nitrazepam, and a number of other benzodiazepines produce age-related changes in pharmacodynamics (Castleden et al. 1977; Reidenberg et al. 1978; Swift et al. 1981; Overstall 1982). An altered receptor-effect relationship has also been found for the opiate derivatives fentanyl and alfentanil (Scott and Stanski 1987), as older patients often show an increased sensitivity to these two narcotics.

4 Practical Aspects in Performing Clinical Trials in Elderly Subjects

Clinical pharmacological trials in the elderly differ in some respects from comparable studies in younger subjects. From the practical point of view, the following points should be taken into consideration when planning and conducting such studies.

4.1 Recruitment of Subjects

When recruiting young healthy subjects, approximately 30 persons must generally be prescreened to arrive at 24 eligible subjects. This number is considerably higher for elderly subjects, i.e., at least 60. An initial check usually reveals anamnestic or clinical signs and symptoms which preclude the assessment "healthy elderly subject" in one-third of this number (20/60), and thus about 40 are suitable for a comprehensive screening investigation (compared with 28 among 30 young potential participants).

The most prevalent exclusion criteria are operations on the gastrointestinal tract or gall bladder, evidence of clinically relevant diseases (hypertension, diabetes mellitus, coronary heart disease, various allergies), and concomitant medications, for which there are frequently no adequate explanations. In around 20% of elderly subjects relevant findings come to light only after contacting the family physician, i.e., the findings were either not mentioned or were played down considerably (epileptic fits, hypertensive crises). It is therefore important that the family doctor be consulted.

In the actual medical screening for inclusion, 10 of the remaining 40 elderly subjects present with clinical, blood chemistry, or hematological findings which preclude participation in the study. These are primarily pathological ECG findings (arrhythmias, AV blocks of the second or third degree, and ST suppression), acute symptoms of a previously undetected illness (in particular high blood pressure and bronchopulmonal diseases), and pathological laboratory values (transaminases, cholesterol, fasting glucose, RBC). Furthermore, up to 20% of potential participants lie above the 20% weight range of the Metropolitan Life Insurance tables. Of the remaining 30 subjects who prove eligible in the prestudy examination (performed around 7 days before study begin), up to four present with symptoms of an acute disease on the morning of the first trial day which exclude them from further participation in the study (once again primarily blood pressure values violating the inclusion criteria, pectanginous complaints, ECG changes, acute bronchitides). It is therefore vital that a thorough clinical investigation be performed immediately before medication by an experienced physician.

4.2 Performance of the Study

When planning a study it must be taken into account that clinical examinations of elderly subjects take much longer than in younger subjects. Therefore the individual measurement times, indeed all scheduled investigations, should not follow in too close chronological proximity, as elderly subjects need considerably more time for various activities than do younger subjects (e.g., dressing and undressing) and require more frequent and longer instructions from the study team. This also applies when specific tests must be extensively explained and trained during the prestudy examinations. This is particularly true if examinations must be performed in a number of different locations (e.g., ECG laboratory, EEG laboratory, laboratory for psychometric measurements). Such a statement may sound trivial, but even experienced investigators have been known to break this basic rule when planning clinical pharmacological trials in elderly subjects. The injudicious practice of "packing" the study with different examinations inevitably leads to misfortune in studies with elderly subjects, as the examination times can be delayed to such an extent that a correct interpretation of the study results is almost impossible.

4.3 Safety Aspects

At the same time, the net of safety examinations (physical examinations, blood pressure measurements, assessment of signs and symptoms, and ECG recordings) performed in the course of the study must be drawn more tightly for elderly subjects than in trials with young subjects. It must be remembered that elderly subjects often report adverse events less frequently and rate them less severely than younger subjects (with the same dose of the study drug), while on the other hand elderly patients in everyday clinical practice tend to report more frequent and more severe adverse reactions than young patients. This underlines the difference between "elderly subjects" and "elderly patients." From a practical point of view, the frequency of adverse events reported in the course of a phase I trial in elderly subjects has therefore little predictive value for the risk assessment. This important caveat with regard to the subjects' safety also must apply to pharmacodynamic variables such as blood pressure measurements. In general, elderly subjects tolerate relatively high doses of a study drug up to a point, but then suddenly show prolonged and intense adverse reactions and pharmacodynamic effects after only a slight dose increase. These in turn can endanger the elderly subject more than a younger participant, considering the restricted functional reserves of persons aged over 50 years. For instance, young subjects can generally tolerate an acute drop in systolic blood pressure of 15–20 mmHg without any relevant problem, while in the elderly it can lead to a dangerous decrease in the supply of blood to vital organs.

Therefore, before a drug is applied in clinical trials in the elderly its clinical pharmacological profile should first be known from studies in young subjects. If the drug is intended for sole therapeutic use in the elderly (thus making studies in young subjects not meaningful), dose increases in the elderly must be implemented with utmost caution. Determination of the maximal tolerated doses, an appropriate step in young subjects to describe the clinical pharmacological profile of a substance and to evaluate the risk-benefit relationship, is not justifiable in elderly subjects due to the increased risks involved.

Instead of dosing the entire group of subjects within a short period, it has proven useful to stagger the medication times over a period of 1 to 2 h to allow sufficient time for an intensive medical care of the subjects and possible emergency measures.

4.4 Sample Size

As the inter- and intraindividual variance of many pharmacodynamic parameters is greater in elderly subjects than in young persons, and as the risk of nonresponders or subjects with excessive reactions is higher, calling for more intensive medical surveillance, sample sizes in studies with elderly subjects should be larger than with young subjects to permit a reliable interpretation of results.

In many clinical pharmacological trials, particularly those with the target parameters "tolerance and safety," the sample size is based on empirical considerations. This is particularly the case in early phase I trials with ascending doses of an investigational drug, and it can be stated that the minimum number of subjects per dose group needed to permit a representative statement is eight to ten. A study design in which new subjects are recruited to each dose group is not recommended since the variability of baseline data is greater in elderly subjects than in younger persons. On the other hand, such a design would have the advantage of minimizing the amount of blood taken per subject, an important consideration in studies in the elderly. One suitable compromise is a study design with two subject groups which alternatively receive the next highest dose.

4.5 Compliance of Subjects with Medication and Study Regulations

If they have been carefully informed about the purpose of the clinical trial and the necessity of regular drug intake, elderly subjects are more reliable than younger subjects in compliance with medication intake — provided they remember. Systems that automatically document medication are less useful than an appropriate and simple packing of medication: individual packs for each medication or study day have proved useful here. Wording on the labels must be in large print and take into account the subjects' potentially poor eyesight. Removing the medication from the pack must be made as simple as possible because many elderly subjects have difficulties with blister packs, for instance.

The majority of clinical pharmacological measurements conducted during a clinical trial with elderly subjects do not differ from those in young subjects; however, the following should be taken into account:

1. As elderly subjects frequently have poor veins, large-volume cannulas should be used to prevent frequent subsequent puncturing of smaller veins, which can cause considerable delays and is fairly unpleasant for the subject. It is also true in clinical pharmacology that a patient or subject judges a physician not on the basis of his medical know-how but on his ability to perform simple tasks. After removing the cannula a pressurized bandage should always be applied to reduce the risk of hematomas, which subjects always regard as very tiresome.

2. During pharmacokinetic examinations subjects should not have to go longer than 2 to 3 h without food, as this can increase the frequency of situation-dependent adverse events.

3. In the exercise ECG many elderly subjects do not achieve a sufficient workload because of rapid muscular exhaustion due to insufficient training. Therefore a study with elderly subjects should be designed so that the work rate increases progressively but has no "increments" such as the ramp test. To assure a reproducible response to exercise (i.e., peak oxygen uptake on two exercise tests on two separate days at the same time of the day 10%) at least two additional exercise tests should be performed for habituation purposes before the start of a study. Subjects with incomplete left bundle branch block (which is not generally an exclusion criterion in clinical trials in the elderly) should be excluded from exercise testing.

4. Compared with the young, elderly subjects have more sensitive skin, thus calling for appropriate skin care during, for instance, repeated 24-h ECG examinations or 24-h blood pressure monitoring.

5. Most psychometric tests were originally developed to record drug effects in young subjects or geriatric patients and can raise problems when applied to healthy elderly subjects, with regard to either the test instructions or the tests themselves. The instructions must be more detailed and given more slowly than for young subjects. This is to ensure that the subject understands the test and to allay anxiety about the unfamiliar task. For instance, it is sufficient to explain a simple critical flicker fusion test just once to young subjects before starting, while elderly subjects must be given instructions before each trial run. When training psychometric tests, it should be remembered that even healthy elderly subjects can tire quickly, and that several short training sessions are therefore preferable.

As to the actual implementation of the tests, it should be considered that elderly subjects can have poor eyesight and hearing and impaired motoricity (test materials with large, high-contrast pictures, no acoustic signals in the high-frequency range).

Regarding speed-oriented tests (reaction time recordings, tracking, memory scans) the variables of inspection time, pacing of task presentation, and time allowed for a response must be adapted to the age group in question. In the absence of published reference ranges for healthy elderly subjects it is advisable first to conduct a pilot study to determine the target level of difficulty for a particular group of elderly subjects. This is the only way to avoid floor effects (i.e., all subjects have scores in the low range), ceiling effects (i.e., all subject have maximum scores), or completely nonsensical results due to excessive demands (resulting in random responses by elderly subjects , while young subjects would normally break off a test, indicating that the test is too difficult).

5 Experimental Findings in Elderly Subjects

The data presented in this volume derive from healthy subjects who participated in phase I studies performed by the authors (H.-P. Breuel, S. Bondy, and P.R. Heine) as principal investigators from 1990 to mid-1992 at the AFB-Klinische Pharmakologie and thereafter at Pharmacon Research in Berlin. All studies had virtually uniform inclusion and exclusion criteria, and all examinations were performed using the same methods. Data from the prestudy screening examination served exclusively to determine subject eligibility and are not considered here. Instead, only the data of the subsequent study day have been entered, even if some parameters were shown to differ between the two days. Baseline values for all subjects are the values measured before medication, and data on variations of different parameters in the course of the study day or during the study were derived solely from subjects under placebo.

5.1 Method

5.1.1 Inclusion Criteria

The following general criteria applied to all subjects (prestudy examination: up to 2 weeks before start of study):

1. Elderly subjects: white, male and female, aged 50 to 80 years; young subjects: white, male, aged 20 to 39 years
2. Normal case history
3. Body weight 55 to 94 kg and within 20% of the recommended range in the Metropolitan Life Insurance tables
4. No relevant findings in the physical examination
5. Systolic blood pressure in supine position (after 3 min rest) between 180 and 100 mmHg, diastolic blood pressure between 100 and 60 mmHg
6. ECG: young subjects: normal ECG (at rest); elderly subjects: normal ECG (at rest) or only mild repolarization disturbances, only AV block of first degree, QRS < 120 ms, only isolated extrasystoles
7. Laboratory results within the reference range or isolated findings without clinical relevance
8. No comedication
9. Nonsmokers or only moderate smokers (up to 10 cigarettes per day)
10. Negative testing for HIV and HBsAg

11. Negative drug screening in urine (cannabinoids, morphine and morphine derivates, amphetamines, barbiturates, benzodiazepenes)

5.1.2 Exclusion Criteria

The following findings/symptoms excluded a subject automatically from participation in the study:
1. Participation in another clinical study within 3 months before start of the trial
2. Known allergic reactions
3. Anamnestic findings of major internal, neurological or psychiatric diseases, or repeated loss of consciousness
4. History of asthmatic or chronic obstructive pulmonary disease,
5. Regular use of alcohol
6. Pathological ECG changes, e.g., AV block of second or higher degree, QRS duration > 120 ms, or QTc > 450 ms
9. Any other abnormality of clinical chemistry, hematology or urinalysis, blood pressure, or ECG

5.1.3 Technical Methods

Blood Pressure Monitoring. Measurements of blood pressure were made from the left arm after the subject had been in a supine position for 3 min and after standing for 2 min. The measurements were conducted using a manual sphygmomanometer and a stethoscope following the method of Riva-Rocci and Korotkoff. The peripheral pulse was taken after 1-min palpation of the radial artery in the left arm.

24-h Blood Pressure Monitoring. The monitoring of 24-h blood pressure was performed after intensive instructions to the subject with a SpaceLabs ABP Monitor model 90202. Measurement intervals were 30 min from 8:00 a.m. to 8:00 p.m. and 60 min from 8:00 p.m. to 8:00 a.m. Registration began between 7:00 and 8:00 a.m. After the end of monitoring (next morning), data were analyzed immediately.

ECG. Twelve-lead ECGs were recorded while the subject was resting in a supine position. Six limb leads as specified by Einthoven (leads I, II, III) and Goldberger (aVR, aVL, aVF) and six precordial leads (V1–V6) according to Wilson were used. A minimum of ten ECG complexes were recorded and documented at a chart speed of 50 mm/s. Lead II was used to assess the ECG times. All ECG times were evaluated by an experienced physician and never automatically (although this would have been technically possible).

24-h ECG. A long-term ECG was recorded for a period of 24 h. Five bipolar leads were positioned on the subjects chest after careful preparation of the skin as follows:

V1: Second right rib, parasternal
V2: Second left rib, parasternal
V3: Fifth right rib, parasternal
V4: Seventh right rib, medioclavicular
V5: Sixth left rib, medioclavicular

ECG recording was started in the morning between 8:00 and 9:00 a.m. The ECG was recorded with a Micro FD recorder (Kontron instruments), continuously measuring ECG data for 24 h. The data from the recorder were transferred via a PC Interface Module (Model K 15192) to a PC for analysis.

Spirometry. The spirometric measurements were carried out using the Flowscreen (Jäger, mod. no. 780577). The variable for evaluation was the forced expiratory volume in 1 s (FEV1). After normal breathing the subjects were requested to take a deep breath (as deep as possible), followed by maximal forced expiration. The measurements were repeated twice, and the highest value was taken for analysis.

Clinical Chemistry Laboratory. Analysis of clinical chemistry parameters was performed with a Hitachi, model 704, with daily runs of quality controls and additional quality samples after each 20 measurements using the following methods:
- Alkaline phosphatase, LDH, SGOT and SGPT: optimized standard method
- γ-GT: kinetic test at 405 nm
- Total bilirubin: DPD method
- Total protein: biuret method
- Uric acid: PAP method, enzymatic dye test
- Creatinine: Crea/PAP method, enzymatic dye test
- Urea (BUN): kinetic UV test, urease
- Cholesterol: CHOD/Pap method, enzymatic dye test
- Triglycerides: GPO/PAP method
- Glucose: hexokinase/G6P-DH
- Sodium, potassium, chloride: ion-selective method

The analytical within-run variations, calculated as the coefficient of variation (CV) using test samples with high and low concentrations, were markedly below 1.5%. Blood samples were taken in supine position without compressing the vein using a large indwelling canulla and nonsiliconized lubricated glass tubes (Vacutainers, Becton-Dickinson) with inert barrier material and clot activator or with plastic tubes (Monovettes, Sarstedt) containing beads for serum separation. After clotting and centrifugation of samples, the serum was analyzed within 24 h.

Hematology. Analysis of hematological parameters was performed with a coulter counter (leukocytes, erythrocytes, hematocrit, thrombocytes), microscopic differentiation with Leukodiff or photometric analysis (hemoglobin). Quick's test was performed with a Coag-A-Mate. Blood samples were taken using siliconized tubes containing 15% potassium EDTA (Monovettes or Vacutainers). Glass tubes containing 3.8% buffered sodium citrate (Vacutainers) were used for taking blood samples for the determination of thromboplastin time (Quick's test).

Adverse Events. The subjects were asked prior to medication by a nonleading question "How do you feel?" The answers were recorded immediately on record forms. Adverse events were graded as follows:
- Mild: signs or symptoms, usually transient, requiring no treatment and generally not interfering with usual activities
- Moderate: signs or symptoms which may be ameliorated by simple therapeutic measures and which may interfere with the usual activities.
- Severe: signs or symptoms which are sufficiently incapacitating that the subject is unable to work or to perform the usual activities, and which may not be ameliorated by simple therapeutic measures.

5.1.4 Data Management and Statistics

The study data of all subjects were originally stored as dbase files. After uniform designation of all variables used in the different studies, the data were converted to variable-specific Excel files using Excel 4.0 and QE (Microsoft). The descriptive statistical analysis was carried out using Excel 4.0, while confirmative statistics were done with SPSS and SAS. The reference range was defined as the 95% range between the 2.5 and 97.5 percentiles. In case of repeated measurements the 95% range of deviations from the baseline value was calculated.

In addition, the critical differences at the 5% level of significance were calculated according to Lienert (1969) as:

$$D_{crit(0.05)} = Z_{(0.05)} \times SD \times \sqrt{2(1-r)}$$

where Z(0.05) denotes the cumulative probability of the standard normal distribution (in case of 5% level: 1.96), SD the standard deviation of the measurement value distribution, and r the correlation coefficient between two consecutive measurements as an estimation of the reliability of the measurement. This definition of Dcrit using the terminology of classical psychometric theory of reliability of measurements can also be expressed in terms of within- and between-subjects variance, which are more popular in the current literature on laboratory methodology (e.g., Gräsbeck and Ahlström 1981). The critical difference Dcrit is the minimal required difference that indicates a statistically significant change (at the 5% level of significance) in consecutive measurements in the same individual. It indicates the limits for a reliably detectable change, taking into account measurement errors of various sources and physiological variation. Changes exceeding the critical difference may be clinically relevant or not (but are at least conspicuous), changes within the critical difference remain below the threshold of discriminability and should be considered as random variation (methodological errors, biological variations). For further details of calculating critical differences, see Lienert (1969) and Weyer (1992).

5.2 Experimental Data

5.2.1 Blood Pressure and Pulse Rate

5.2.1.1 Baseline Values

Supine Position

Table 13. Supine systolic blood pressure (mmHg), healthy subjects (8:00–9:00 A.M.)

Population	n	Mean ± SD	Median	Reference range
Men, 20–39 years	1265	119.1 ± 10.5	120	100–142
20–29 years	900	119.4 ± 10.5	120	100–142
30–39 years	365	118.4 ± 10.3	118	100–140
Men and women 50–80 years	1187	129.4 ± 17.4	128	100–168
50–59 years	311	121.8 ± 15.9	118	98–160
60–69 years	652	129.8 ± 16.4	129	100–164
70–80 years	224	138.8 ± 17.6	138	106–172
Men, 50–80 years	551	129.2 ± 16.7	128	100–162
Women, 50–80 years	636	129.6 ± 18.0	128	100–168

Table 14. Supine diastolic blood pressure (mmHg), healthy subjects (8:00–9:00 A.M.)

Population	n	Mean ± SD	Median	Reference range
Men, 20–39 years	1265	73.8 ± 7.7	72	60–90
20–29 years	900	73.5 ± 7.6	72	60–90
30–39 years	365	74.4 ± 7.9	74	60–90
Men and women, 50–80 years	1187	78.9 ± 9.5	80	60–98
50–59 years	311	77.5 ± 9.5	78	60–98
60–69 years	652	79.4 ± 9.2	80	60–98
70–80 years	224	79.7 ± 10.2	80	62–100
Men, 50–80 years	551	79.6 ± 9.3	80	64–98
Women, 50–80 years	636	78.3 ± 9.7	78	60–98

Table 15. Supine pulse rate (bpm), healthy subjects (8:00–9:00 A.M.)

Population	n	Mean ± SD	Median	Reference range
Men, 20–39 years	1265	65.2 ± 8.8	64	50–84
20–29 years	900	65.2 ± 8.8	64	50–85
30–39 years	365	65.2 ± 8.6	64	48–83
Men and women, 50–80 years	1187	68.9 ± 9.1	68	52–88
50–59 years	311	68.3 ± 8.6	68	55–88
60–69 years	652	68.4 ± 9.2	68	52–88
70–80 years	224	71.0 ± 9.4	71	52–89
Men, 50–80 years	551	67.8 ± 8.8	68	52–87
Women, 50–80 years	636	69.8 ± 9.3	68	54–91

Standing Position

Table 16. Systolic blood pressure (mmHg) after 3-min standing, healthy subjects (8:00–9:00 A.M.)

Population	n	Mean ± SD	Median	Reference range
Men, 20–39 years	757	117.3 ± 10.7	116	100–142
20–29 years	550	117.4 ± 10.1	118	100–138
30–39 years	207	117.1 ± 12.2	116	98–144
Men and women, 50–80 years	1050	127.8 ± 17.6	126	98–168
50–59 years	243	121.1 ± 16.9	120	96–168
60–69 years	587	127.3 ± 16.8	126	100–150
70–80 years	220	136.6 ± 16.8	138	104–174
Men, 50–80 years	536	127.5 ± 17.4	126	98–168
Women, 50–80 years	514	128.1 ± 17.7	126	98–168

Table 17. Diastolic blood pressure (mmHg) after 3-min standing, healthy subjects (8:00–9:00 A.M.)

Population	n	Mean ± SD	Median	Reference range
Men, 20–39 years	757	77.3 ± 8.3	78	62–98
20–29 years	550	77.3 ± 8.1	78	62–92
30–39 years	207	77.5 ± 9.0	78	60–98
Men and women, 50–80 years	1050	81.5 ± 10.1	80	60–102
50–59 years	243	80.4 ± 10.6	80	60–100
60–69 years	587	82.0 ± 10.0	80	62–96
70–80 years	220	81.8 ± 9.5	80	64–102
Men, 50–80 years	536	82.1 ± 9.8	81	62–102
Women, 50–80 years	514	81.0 ± 10.3	80	60–102

Table 18. Pulse rate (bpm) after 3-min standing, healthy subjects (8:00–9:00 A.M.)

Population	n	Mean ± SD	Median	Reference range
Men, 20–39 years	757	77.8 ± 10.4	76	60–100
20–29 years	550	78.2 ± 10.6	78	60–98
30–39 years	207	76.5 ± 9.9	75	60–96
Men and women, 50–80 years	1050	76.4 ± 10.2	76	60–98
50–59 years	243	75.0 ± 9.8	74	60–96
60–69 years	587	75.9 ± 10.1	76	59–95
70–80 years	220	79.3 ± 10.6	80	58–100
Men, 50–80 years	536	76.4 ± 10.2	76	59–98
Women, 50–80 years	514	76.5 ± 10.3	76	60–98

Orthostatic Reaction

Table 19. Differences of systolic blood pressure (mmHg) in supine position and after 3-min standing, (standing-supine), healthy subjects (8:00–9:00 A.M.)

Population	*n*	Mean ± SD	Median	Reference range
Men, 20–39 years	757	–2.8 ± 7.6	–2	–18 to 12
20–29 years	550	–2.9 ± 7.5	–4	–18 to 10
30–39 years	207	–2.6 ± 7.9	–2	–18 to 14
Men and women, 50–80 years	1050	–2.5 ± 10.8	–2	–26 to 20
50–59 years	243	–2.3 ± 9.5	–2	–20 to 18
60–69 years	587	–2.6 ± 10.9	–2	–26 to 10
70–80 years	220	–2.7 ± 12.1	–3	–28 to 20
Men, 50–80 years	536	–1.6 ± 10.5	–2	–24 to 22
Women, 50–80 years	514	–3.5 ± 11.1	–4	–28 to 20

Table 20. Differences of diastolic blood pressure (mmHg) in supine position and after 3-min standing, (standing-supine), healthy subjects (8:00–9:00 A.M.)

Population	*n*	Mean ± SD	Median	Reference range
Men, 20–39 years	757	3.9 ± 7.1	4	–10 to 18
20–29 years	550	4.1 ± 7.0	4	– 8 to 18
30–39 years	207	3.6 ± 7.4	4	–10 to 22
Men and women, 50–80 years	1050	2.3 ± 7.2	2	–12 to 20
50–59 years	243	2.1 ± 6.5	2	–12 to 14
60–69 years	587	2.5 ± 7.1	2	–12 to 12
70–80 years	220	2.0 ± 8.0	2	–16 to 18
Men, 50–80 years	536	2.4 ± 7.2	2	–12 to 18
Women, 50–80 years	514	2.3 ± 7.2	2	–12 to 18

Table 21. Differences in pulse rate (bpm) in supine position and after 3-min standing, (standing-supine), healthy subjects (8:00–9:00 A.M.)

Population	*n*	Mean ± SD	Median	Reference range
Men, 20–39 years	757	12.6 ± 9.0	10	–2 to 33
20–29 years	550	12.9 ± 9.3	12	–2 to 31
30–39 years	207	11.7 ± 8.0	9	0 to 33
Men and women, 50–80 years	1050	8.1 ± 7.5	8	–7 to 25
50–59 years	243	8.1 ± 7.3	8	–8 to 17
60–69 years	587	7.9 ± 7.2	8	–7 to 17
70–80 years	220	8.4 ± 8.4	7	–5 to 30
Men, 50–80 years	536	8.5 ± 6.9	8	–6 to 23
Women, 50–80 years	514	7.6 ± 8.1	7	–7 to 25

5.2.1.2 Changes in Blood Pressure and Pulse Rate During Study Day

Elderly Subjects

Table 22. Differences from baseline in systolic and diastolic blood pressure (mmHg) and pulse rate (bpm) in supine position during study day, in healthy men and women aged 50 to 80 years (baseline 8:00–9:00 A.M.)

Time after first measurement	n	Mean ± SD	95% diff.[a]	D_{crit}
2 h				
Systolic BP	141	0.21 ± 12.30	−22 to 24	25.7
Diastolic BP	141	−1.45 ± 8.35	−16 to 14	16.1
Pulse rate	141	−2.31 ± 8.49	−20 to 12	16.4
4 h				
Systolic BP	210	−0.94 ± 12.29	−24 to 20	23.8
Diastolic BP	210	−1.11 ± 9.21	−20 to 18	18.0
Pulse rate	210	−1.06 ± 9.37	−18 to 16	18.4
6 h				
Systolic BP	168	−2.18 ± 11.92	−22 to 22	23.0
Diastolic BP	168	−4.16 ± 9.45	−24 to 14	18.8
Pulse rate	168	3.26 ± 10.78	−21 to 23	21.4
10 h				
Systolic BP	128	−1.16 ± 12.54	−26 to 22	23.5
Diastolic BP	128	−2.21 ± 10.56	−24 to 18	20.3
Pulse rate	128	2.48 ± 10.01	−16 to 18	22.7

[a] 95% range of differences from baseline.

Young Subjects

Table 23. Differences from baseline in systolic and diastolic blood pressure (mmHg) and pulse rate (bpm) in supine position during study day in healthy men and women aged 20–39 years (baseline 8:00–9:00 A.M.)

Time after first measurement	n	Mean ± SD	95% diff.[a]	D_{crit}
2 h				
Systolic BP	287	−1.16 ± 5.58	−10 to 10	12.8
Diastolic BP	287	0.40 ± 6.03	−12 to 12	10.7
Pulse rate	287	−2.92 ± 7.19	−19 to 10	11.5
4 h				
Systolic BP	233	0.94 ± 6.76	−12 to 14	14.5
Diastolic BP	233	−0.22 ± 6.03	−10 to 12	11.9
Pulse rate	233	1.69 ± 8.45	−14 to 19	16.8
6 h				
Systolic BP	254	0.24 ± 7.31	−12 to 16	10.6
Diastolic BP	254	−1.55 ± 6.39	−12 to 12	13.0
Pulse rate	254	0.98 ± 7.32	−12 to 15	14.0
10 h				
Systolic BP	226	2.08 ± 7.69	−12 to 16	17.0
Diastolic BP	226	−1.16 ± 6.13	−12 to 12	13.1
Pulse rate	226	2.19 ± 7.43	−12 to 16	15.0

[a] 95% range of differences from baseline.

5.2.1.3 Changes in Blood Pressure and Pulse Rate After Repeated Measurements

Table 24. Changes in systolic and diastolic blood pressure (mmHg) and pulse rate (bpm) in supine position after 24 and 48 h, healthy subjects, differences from baseline, (baseline 8:00–9:00 A.M.)

Population	n	Mean ± SD	95% diff.[a]	D_{crit}
Changes after 24 h				
Men, 20–39 years				
Systolic BP	144	2.3 ± 5.0	−8 to 10	10.0
Diastolic BP	144	0.5 ± 4.0	−8 to 8	7.7
Pulse rate	144	0.3 ± 6.1	−12 to 9	12.8
Men and women, 50–80 years				
Systolic BP	180	0.4 ± 3.4	−6 to 6	6.6
Diastolic BP	180	−0.5 ± 4.0	−8 to 8	7.1
Pulse rate	180	0.0 ± 4.6	−8 to 11	8.5
Changes after 48 h				
Men and women, 50–80 years				
Systolic BP	123	1.9 ± 9.9	−14 to 20	18.0
Diastolic BP	123	−1.1 ± 8.6	−16 to 16	15.8
Pulse rate	123	0.0 ± 8.1	−17 to 16	16.2

[a] 95% range of differences from baseline.

Table 25. Changes in supine systolic and diastolic blood pressure (mmHg) and pulse rate (bpm) after 1 week, differences from baseline, healthy subjects (baseline 8:00–9:00 A.M.)

Population	n	Mean ± SD	95% diff.[a]	D_{crit}
Men, 20–39 years				
Systolic BP	95	0.62 ± 3.32	−4 to 8	6.2
Diastolic BP	95	0.16 ± 3.32	−6 to 8	6.6
Pulse rate	95	−0.19 ± 6.01	−10 to 12	10.8
Men and women, 50–80 years				
Systolic BP	229	−0.83 ± 7.15	−12 to 13	13.6
Diastolic BP	229	−1.34 ± 5.88	12 to 10	11.5
Pulse rate	229	−1.38 ± 9.67	−16 to 16	18.1

Table 26. Changes in supine systolic and diastolic blood pressure (mmHg) and pulse rate (bpm) after 2 and 3 weeks, differences from baseline, healthy subjects aged 50–80 years (baseline 8:00–9:00 A.M.)

Population	n	Mean ± SD	95% diff.[a]	D_{crit}
2 Weeks				
Men and women, 50–80 years				
Systolic BP	211	−1.00 ± 8.59	−15 to 14	16.4
Diastolic BP	211	−0.49 ± 8.63	−14 to 18	16.9
Pulse rate	211	0.14 ± 10.26	−22 to 22	20.1
3 Weeks				
Men and women, 50–80 years				
Systolic BP	246	−0.09 ± 7.94	−14 to 16	15.2
Diastolic BP	246	0.30 ± 7.39	−14 to 14	14.1
Pulse rate	246	0.13 ± 8.52	−18 to 18	16.6

[a] 95% range of differences from baseline.

5.2.1.4 Confirmative Statistics of Blood Pressure Findings

Baseline Values

Table 27. Comparison of differences in baseline blood pressures and pulse rates of selected subject groups: statistical significance

	Elderly men vs. young men	Elderly men vs. elderly women	50–59 years vs. 60–69 years	50–59 years vs. 70–80 years	60–69 years vs. 70–80 years	30–39 years vs. 50–59 years, men	20–29 years vs. 30–39 years
Supine							
Systolic BP	++	ns	++	++	++	+	+
Diastolic BP	++	ns	+	ns	ns	++	ns
Pulse rate	++	++	ns	++	++	ns	ns
Standing							
Systolic BP	++	ns	++	++	++	ns	ns
Diastolic BP	++	ns	ns	ns	ns	++	ns
Pulse rate	+	ns	ns	++	++	+	ns
Diff. standing-supine							
Systolic BP	+	ns	ns	ns	ns	ns	ns
Diastolic BP	++	ns	ns	ns	ns	ns	ns
Pulse rate	++	ns	ns	ns	ns	+	+

++, $p \leq 0.01$; +, $p \leq 0.05$; ns, not significant (two-tailed p values, Mann-Whitney U–Wilcoxon rank sum W test).

REPEATED MEASUREMENTS

Table 28. Comparison of differences in blood pressures and pulse rates during study day: statistical significance

	2 h	4 h	6 h	10 h
Elderly subjects				
Supine				
Systolic BP	ns	ns	++	ns
Diastolic BP	ns	+	++	+
Pulse rate	++	++	++	++
Standing				
Systolic BP	ns	ns	+	ns
Diastolic BP	+	ns	++	+
Pulse rate	++	ns	ns	++
Young subjects				
Supine				
Systolic BP	++	+	ns	++
Diastolic BP	ns	ns	++	++
Pulse rate	++	++	+	++

++, $p \leq 0.01$; +, $p \leq 0.05$; ns, not significant (versus baseline, two-tailed p values, Wilcoxon matched-pairs signed-rank test).

Table 29. Comparison of differences in blood pressures and pulse rates on different study days: statistical significance

	24 h	48 h	1 Week	2 Weeks	3 Weeks
Elderly subjects					
Supine					
Systolic BP	ns	ns	ns	ns	ns
Diastolic BP	ns	ns	+	ns	ns
Pulse rate	ns	ns	ns	ns	ns
Standing					
Systolic BP	ns	ns	+	ns	+
Diastolic BP	ns	+	ns	ns	ns
Pulse rate	ns	ns	ns	ns	ns
Young subjects					
Supine					
Systolic BP	++	−	ns	−	−
Diastolic BP	ns	−	ns	−	−
Pulse rate	ns	−	ns	−	−

++, $p \leq 0.01$; +, $p \leq 0.05$; ns, not significant (versus baseline, two-tailed p values, Wilcoxon matched-pairs signed-rank test).

Table 30. Comparison of differences in blood pressures and pulse rates between elderly and young subjects after 24 h and 1 week: statistical significance

	24 H	1 Week
Systolic BP	++	+
Diastolic BP	+	+
Pulse rate of	ns	+

++, $p \leq 0.01$; +, $p \leq 0.05$; ns, not significant (two-tailed p values, Mann-Whitney U–Wilcoxon rank sum W test).

5.2.2 Ambulatory Blood Pressure Monitoring

5.2.2.1 Baseline Values

Table 31. Ambulatory blood pressure monitoring in normotensive and hypertensive subjects, men and women aged 50–80 years (start of registration between 7:00 and 8:00 A.M.)

	n	Mean ± SD	Median	Reference range[a], 2.5/97.5 percentile[b]
Normotensives				
Systolic BP				
24-h period	309	125.3 ± 10.8	126	107 –145
Day period	309	129.4 ± 11.2	130	110 –150
Night period	309	119.4 ± 11.7	120	97 –144
Diastolic BP				
24-h period	309	75.6 ± 6.7	75	63 –88
Day period	309	79.3 ± 7.1	80	66 –92
Night period	309	70.3 ± 7.2	71	57 –84
Hypertensives				
Systolic BP				
24-h period	157	152.7 ± 12.8	151	129.7/179.9
Day period	157	159.1 ± 12.9	157	136.9/187.5
Night period	157	144.9 ± 14.2	144	119.7/174.2
Diastolic BP				
24-h period	157	97.3 ± 7.6	96	85.4/109.5
Day period	157	108.0 ± 6.1	107	98.5/119.0
Night period	157	89.9 ± 8.7	89	76.2/102.6

[a] Values for normotensives.

[b] Values for hypertensives.

5.2.2.2 Course of Blood Pressure During Study Day

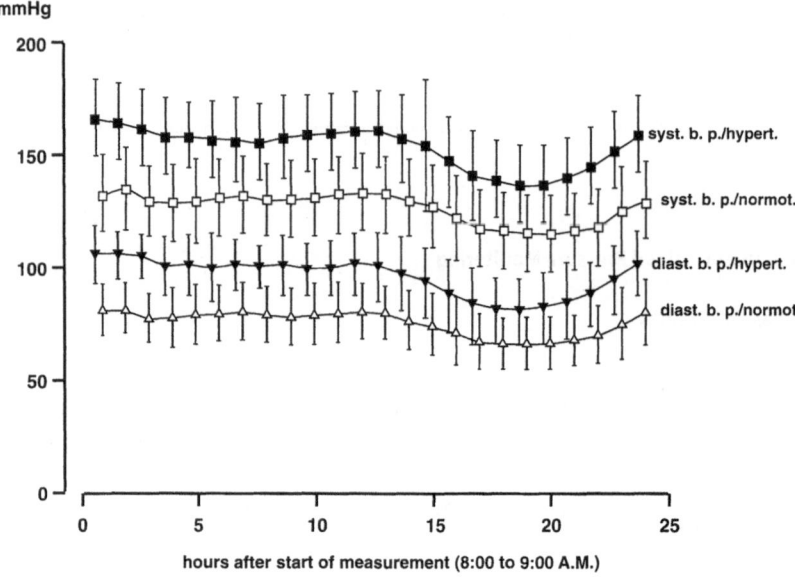

Fig. 5. Systolic and diastolic blood pressure in 211 healthy, normotensive subjects aged 50–80 years and in 142 hypertensive subjects aged 50–80 years: 24-h blood pressure monitoring, mean ± SD

5.2.2.3 Changes After 2 Weeks

Table 32. Ambulatory blood pressure monitoring: differences (mmHg) from baseline systolic and diastolic blood pressure after 2 weeks (± 2 days), normotensive subjects aged 50–80 years (start of registration between 7:00 and 8:00 A.M.)

	n	Mean ± SD	95% diff.[a]	D_{crit}
Systolic BP				
24-h period	101	−0.6 ± 4.8	−8 to 8	9.6
Day period	101	−0.9 ± 4.6	−8 to 8	9.3
Night period	101	0.1 ± 6.2	−10 to 10	12.6
Diastolic BP				
24-h period	101	−1.0 ± 4.2	−8 to 7	8.4
Day period	101	−0.7 ± 4.1	−8 to 8	8.4
Night period	101	0.1 ± 6.0	−9 to 13	12.1

[a] 95% range of differences from baseline.

5.2.2.4 Confirmatory Statistics of 24-h Blood Pressure Findings

Table 33. Comparison of mean differences in 24-h blood pressure recordings, normotensive and hypertensive subjects

	Normotensives vs. hypertensives*	Normotensives: baseline vs. 2 weeks**
24-h period		
Systolic BP	++	ns
Diastolic BP	++	ns
Day period		
Systolic BP	++	ns
Diastolic BP	++	ns
Night period		
Systolic BP	++	ns
Diastolic BP	++	ns

++, $p \leq 0.01$; *ns*, not significant (two-tailed *p*-values, *Mann-Whitney U-Wilcoxon rank sum W test, **Wilcoxon matched-pairs signed-rank test; for *n*: see Tables 31 and 32)).

5.2.3 ECG Times

5.2.3.1 Baseline Values of ECG Times

Table 34. RR time (s), healthy subjects (8:00–9:00 A.M.)

Population	n	Mean ± SD	Median	Reference range
Men, 20–39 years	547	1.01 ± 0.15	1.00	0.73–1.30
Men and women, 50–80 years	655	0.94 ± 0.13	0.93	0.69–1.19
50–59 years	264	0.91 ± 0.12	0.91	0.69–1.18
60–69 years	287	0.95 ± 0.13	0.95	0.69–1.16
70–80 years	104	0.97 ± 0.16	0.95	0.68–1.30
Men, 50–80 years	344	0.96 ± 0.13	0.95	0.73–1.23
Women, 50–80 years	311	0.91 ± 0.13	0.91	0.66–1.16

Table 35. PQ time (s), healthy subjects (8:00–9:00 A.M.)

Population	n	Mean ± SD	Median	Reference range
Men, 20–39 years	1638	0.16 ± 0.02	0.16	0.12–0.20
20–29 years	1053	0.16 ± 0.02	0.16	0.12–0.20
30–39 years	585	0.16 ± 0.02	0.16	0.13–0.20
Men and women, 50–80 years	1198	0.16 ± 0.02	0.16	0.12–0.20
50–59 years	360	0.16 ± 0.02	0.15	0.12–0.20
60–69 years	623	0.17 ± 0.02	0.17	0.13–0.21
70–80 years	215	0.17 ± 0.02	0.16	0.12–0.21
Men, 50–80 years	582	0.16 ± 0.02	0.16	0.13–0.21
Women, 50–80 years	616	0.16 ± 0.02	0.16	0.12–0.20

Table 36. QRS time (s), healthy subjects (8:00–9:00 A.M.)

Population	n	Mean ± SD	Median	Reference range
Men, 20–39 years	1638	0.09 ± 0.01	0.09	0.07–0.11
20–29 years	1053	0.09 ± 0.01	0.09	0.08–0.11
30–39 years	585	0.09 ± 0.01	0.09	0.07–0.12
Men and women, 50–80 years	1197	0.09 ± 0.01	0.09	0.07–0.11
50–59 years	360	0.09 ± 0.01	0.08	0.07–0.10
60–69 years	623	0.09 ± 0.01	0.09	0.07–0.11
70–80 years	214	0.09 ± 0.01	0.09	0.07–0.11
Men, 50–80 years	581	0.09 ± 0.01	0.09	0.07–0.11
Women, 50–80 years	616	0.09 ± 0.01	0.09	0.07–0.11

Table 37. QT time (s), healthy subjects (8:00–9:00 A.M.)

Population	n	Mean ± SD	Median	Reference range
Men, 20–39 years	1638	0.38 ± 0.03	0.38	0.33–0.43
20–29 years	1053	0.38 ± 0.03	0.38	0.33–0.43
30–39 years	585	0.38 ± 0.03	0.38	0.34–0.44
Men and women, 50–80 years	1198	0.39 ± 0.02	0.39	0.35–0.44
50–59 years	360	0.38 ± 0.02	0.38	0.34–0.43
60–69 years	623	0.40 ± 0.02	0.40	0.35–0.44
70–80 years	215	0.40 ± 0.03	0.40	0.35–0.46
Men, 50–80 years	582	0.39 ± 0.02	0.39	0.35–0.44
Women, 50–80 years	616	0.39 ± 0.03	0.40	0.34–0.44

Table 38. QTc time (s), healthy subjects (8:00–9:00 A.M.)

Population	n	Mean ± SD	Median	Reference range
Men, 20–39 years	601	0.39 ± 0.02	0.39	0.34–0.43
Men and Women, 50–80 years	571	0.40 ± 0.02	0.40	0.37–0.44
50–59 years	251	0.40 ± 0.02	0.40	0.37–0.44
60–69 years	246	0.41 ± 0.02	0.40	0.37–0.45
70–80 years	74	0.40 ± 0.02	0.40	0.35–0.43
Men, 50–80 years	298	0.41 ± 0.02	0.41	0.37–0.44
Women, 50–80 years	273	0.40 ± 0.02	0.40	0.36–0.44

Table 39. Heart rate (bpm), healthy subjects (8:00–9:00 A.M.)

Population	n	Mean ± SD	Median	Reference range
Men, 20–39 years	1638	60.6 ± 9.4	61	46–82
Men and women, 50–80 years	1198	65.8 ± 9.5	65	50–87
50–59 years	360	61.8 ± 7.8	61	50–80
60–69 years	623	67.4 ± 9.4	67	51–89
70–80 years	215	67.9 ± 10.1	66	51–90
Men, 50–80 years	582	65.6 ± 8.9	64	52–87
Women, 50–80 years	616	66.0 ± 9.9	66	49–85

5.2.3.2 Changes in ECG Times During Study Day

Table 40. Changes in ECG times during study day, differences from baseline, healthy men and women aged 50–80 years (baseline 8:00–9:00 A.M.)

Time after first measurement	n	Mean ± SD	95% diff.[a]	D_{crit}
2 h				
RR (s)	130	0.05 ± 0.11	–0.21 to 0.26	0.20
PQ (s)	146	0.00 ± 0.01	–0.02 to 0.02	0.02
QRS (s)	146	0.00 ± 0.03	–0.02 to 0.02	0.02
QT (s)	146	0.01 ± 0.02	–0.03 to 0.04	0.04
Heart rate (bpm)	146	–3.2 ± 7.6	–16 to 17	15.9
4 h				
RR (s)	126	0.01 ± 0.10	–0.21 to 0.20	0.20
PQ (s)	142	0.00 ± 0.01	–0.02 to 0.02	0.02
QRS (s)	142	0.00 ± 0.01	–0.02 to 0.02	0.02
QT (s)	142	0.00 ± 0.02	–0.03 to 0.03	0.03
Heart rate (bpm)	142	–0.9 ± 6.5	–14 to 11	13.5
6 h				
RR (s)	199	-0.04 ± 0.11	–0.27 to 0.19	0.22
PQ (s)	209	0.00 ± 0.01	–0.03 to 0.03	0.03
QRS (s)	209	0.00 ± 0.01	–0.01 to 0.02	0.02
QT (s)	209	0.00 ± 0.02	–0.04 to 0.02	0.03
Heart rate (bpm)	209	2.9 ± 7.4	–12 to 18	15.4
12 h				
RR (s)	69	–0.03 ± 0.10	–0.27 to 0.15	0.21
PQ (s)	85	0.00 ± 0.01	–0.03 to 0.02	0.03
QRS (s)	85	0.00 ± 0.01	–0.01 to 0.02	0.02
QT (s)	85	–0.01 ± 0.02	–0.04 to 0.05	0.04
Heart rate (bpm)	85	2.0 ± 7.0	–10 to 18	14.3

[a] 95% range of differences from baseline.

5.2.3.3 Changes in ECG Times After Repeated Measurements

Table 41. Changes in ECG times and heart rate during repeated measurements, differences from baseline, healthy men and women aged 50–80 years (baseline 8:00–9:00)

Time after first measurement	n	Mean ± SD	95% diff.[a]	D_{crit}
24 h				
RR (s)	180	−0.01 ± 0.09	−0.17 to 0.19	0.19
PQ (s)	186	0.00 ± 0.01	−0.02 to 0.02	0.02
QRS (s)	186	0.00 ± 0.01	−0.02 to 0.01	0.02
QT (s)	186	0.00 ± 0.02	−0.03 to 0.03	0.03
QTc (s)	180	0.00 ± 0.02	−0.03 to 0.03	0.04
Heart rate (bpm)	186	0.5 ± 7.1	−12 to 15	14.3
48 h				
RR (s)	156	−0.01 ± 0.10	−0.22 to 0.15	0.19
PQ (s)	156	0.00 ± 0.01	−0.03 to 0.03	0.03
QRS (s)	156	0.00 ± 0.01	−0.02 to 0.01	0.02
QT (s)	156	0.00 ± 0.02	−0.03 to 0.03	0.03
QTc (s)	156	0.00 ± 0.02	−0.03 to 0.04	0.04
Heart rate (bpm)	156	0.9 ± 7.8	−14 to 15	16.1
1 week				
RR (s)	178	0.01 ± 0.10	−0.21 to 0.22	0.21
PQ (s)	313	0.00 ± 0.01	−0.03 to 0.03	0.03
QRS (s)	313	0.00 ± 0.01	−0.02 to 0.02	0.02
QT (s)	313	0.00 ± 0.02	−0.04 to 0.04	0.05
QTc (s)	178	0.00 ± 0.02	−0.04 to 0.04	0.04
Heart rate (bpm)	302	0.5 ± 7.6	−17 to 13	14.9
2 weeks				
RR (s)	245	0.01 ± 0.10	−0.19 to 0.21	0.20
PQ (s)	280	0.00 ± 0.01	−0.02 to 0.03	0.03
QRS (s)	280	0.00 ± 0.01	−0.02 to 0.02	0.02
QT (s)	280	0.00 ± 0.02	−0.03 to 0.04	0.03
QTc (s)	202	0.00 ± 0.02	−0.04 to 0.03	0.04
Heart rate (bpm)	280	−1.1 ± 7.7	−16 to 14	15.7

[a] 95% range of differences from baseline.

5.2.3.4 Confirmative Statistics

Baseline Values

Table 42. Comparison of ECG times in selected subject groups: statistical significance

	Elderly men vs. young men	Elderly men vs. elderly women	50–59 years vs. 60–69 years	50–59 years vs. 70–80 years	60–69 years vs. 70–80 years	20–29 years vs. 50–59 years, men	30–39 years vs. 50–59 years, men	20–29 years vs. 30–39 years
RR	++	++	++	+	ns	++	++	ns
P	++	++	ns	ns	ns	++	++	ns
PQ	++	ns	++	++	ns	++	ns	++
QRS	++	ns	++	++	ns	++	++	++
QT	++	ns	++	++	ns	++	ns	++
QTc	++	++	ns	ns	ns	++	++	ns

++, $p \leq 0.01$; +, $p \leq 0.05$; ns, not significant (two-tailed p values, Mann-Whitney U–Wilcoxon rank sum W test).

Repeated Measurements

Table 43. Comparison of ECG times during study day, healthy men and women aged 50–80 years: statistical significance

	Baseline vs. 2 h	Baseline vs. 4 h	Baseline vs. 6 h	Baseline vs. 12 h
RR	++	ns	++	ns
PQ	ns	ns	ns	+
QRS	ns	ns	ns	ns
QT	++	ns	++	ns
Heart rate	++	ns	++	ns

++, $p \leq 0.01$; +, $p \leq 0.05$; *ns*, not significant (two-tailed p values, Wilcoxon matched-pairs signed rank test).

Table 44. Comparison of ECG times on different study days, healthy men and women aged 50-80 years: statistical significance

	Baseline vs. 24 h	Baseline vs. 48 h	Baseline vs. 1 week	Baseline vs. 2 weeks
RR	ns	ns	ns	ns
PQ	ns	ns	ns	ns
QRS	ns	ns	ns	ns
QT	ns	ns	ns	ns
QT_c	ns	ns	ns	+
Heart rate	ns	ns	ns	ns

++, $p \leq 0.01$; +, $p \leq 0.05$; *ns*, not significant (two-tailed p values, Wilcoxon matched-pairs signed rank test).

5.2.4 Ambulatory ECG Monitoring

5.2.4.1 Baseline Values

Table 45. Ambulatory 24-h ECG monitoring, men and women aged 50–80 years (start of registration between 8:00 and 9:00 A.M.)

	n	Mean ± SD	Median	Reference range
Heart rate (bpm)				
Men and women	328	74.8 ± 8.1	75	58–91
Men	172	74.8 ± 8.2	75	59–91
Women	156	74.9 ± 7.9	75	58–91
TEPS				
Men and women	328	13.4 ± 22.9	6	0–80
Men	172	12.3 ± 24.9	4	0–85
Women	156	14.6 ± 20.5	9	0–78
BEPS				
Men and women	328	1.3 ± 10.3	0	0–12
Men	172	0.6 ± 2.6	0	0–11
Women	156	2.0 ± 14.7	0	0–16
Pauses				
Men and women	328	6.8 ± 74.7	0	0–11
Men	172	3.3 ± 38.6	0	0–7
Women	156	10.7 ± 100.5	6	0–39
SVE				
Men and women	328	58.3 ± 208.0	8	0–683
Men	172	50.8 ± 173.5	7	0–463
Women	156	66.7 ± 240.7	9	0–683
ISO				
Men and women	328	204.0 ± 559.4	43	1–1201
Men	172	169.2 ± 451.9	47	0–1201
Women	156	242.4 ± 657.3	143	2–1609

TEPS, Tachycardiac episode; *BEPS*, bradicardiac episodes; *SVE*; supraventricular extrasystole; *ISO*, isolated ventricular episode.

5.2.4.2 Changes After Repeated Measurements

Table 46. Changes in 24 h ECG recording after 2 and 3 weeks, differences from baseline, men and women aged 50–80 years

	n	Mean ± SD	95% diff.[a]	D_{crit}
Heart rate (bpm)	168	−0.2 ± 6.8	−13 to 17	13.2
TEPS	168	1.4 ± 23.9	−49 to 55	42.1
BEPS	168	−1.3 ± 14.9	−13 to 5	8.8
Pauses	168	−2.9 ± 24.5	−10 to 11	9.4
SVE	168	3.1 ± 188.2	−360 to 270	332.6
ISO	168	−16.3 ±480.0	−592 to 529	520.8

TEPS, Tachycardiac episode; *BEPS*, bradicardiac episodes; *SVE*; supraventricular extrasystole; *ISO*, isolated ventricular episode.

[a] 95% range of differences from baseline.

5.2.4.3 Confirmatory Statistics

Table 47. Comparison of findings from 24-h ECG monitoring between selected subject groups

	Elderly men vs. elderly women	50 years vs. 60 years	50 years vs 70 years	60 years vs. 70 years	Changes after 2 weeks
Heart rate	ns	ns	++	+	ns
TEPS	++	++	++	++	ns
BEPS	ns	ns	ns	ns	ns
Pauses	ns	ns	ns	ns	ns
SVE	ns	ns	ns	ns	ns
ISO	ns	ns	ns	ns	ns

++, $p \leq 0.01$; +, $p \leq 0.05$; *ns*; not significant (two-tailed p values, Mann-Whitney U–Wilcoxon rank sum W test).

TEPS, Tachycardiac episode; *BEPS*, bradicardiac episodes; *SVE*; supraventricular extrasystole; *ISO*, isolated ventricular episode.

5.2.5 Spirometry (FEV1)

5.2.5.1 Baseline Values

Table 48. Reference ranges for FEV_1, young and elderly subjects (8:00–9:00 A.M.)

Population	n	Mean ± SD	Median	Reference range
Young subjects				
Men				
20–39 years	433	4.57 ± 0.47	4.56	3.7–5.6
20–29 years	294	4.61 ± 0.47	4.60	3.8–5.6
30–39 years	139	4.48 ± 0.46	4.52	3.6–5.2
Elderly subjects				
Men and women				
50–80 years	502	2.71 ± 0.76	2.60	1.4–4.7
50–59 years	102	2.87 ± 0.65	2.76	2.1–4.5
60–69 years	268	2.73 ± 0.79	2.68	1.5–4.8
70–80 years	132	2.55 ± 0.77	2.40	1.3–4.3
Men, 50–80 years	240	3.05 ± 0.78	2.92	2.0–4.8
Women, 50–80 years	262	2.40 ± 0.59	2.36	1.4–3.5

5.2.5.2 Changes During Study Day and After 1 Week

Table 49. Changes from baseline FEV_1 (l) after repeated measurements, elderly men and women aged 50–80 years

Time	n	Mean ± SD	95% diff.[a]	D_{crit}
4 h	251	0.01±0.31	-0.60 to 0.56	0.60
1 week	161	0.01±0.30	-0.80 to 0.84	0.63

[a] 95% range of differences from baseline.

5.2.5.3 Confirmatory Statistics

Table 50. Comparison of baseline values and repeated measurements of FEV1: statistical significance

	p
Baseline values[a]	
20–29 years vs. 30–39 years	ns
20–29 years vs. 50–59 years	++
50–59 years vs. 60–69 years	ns
50–59 years vs. 70–80 years	++
60–69 years vs. 70–80 years	+
Men 20–39 years vs. men 50–80 years	++
Men 50–80 years vs. women 50–80 years	++
Repeated measurements[b]	
Men and women, 50–80 years	
Baseline / 4 h	ns
Baseline / 1 week	ns

++, $p \leq 0.01$; +, $p \leq 0.05$; *ns*, not significant.

[a] Mann-Whitney *U*–Wilcoxon rank sum W test.

[b] Wilcoxon matched-pairs signed-rank test.

5.2.6 Clinical Chemistry

5.2.6.1 Baseline Values

Table 51. Reference ranges for alkaline phosphatase (U/l), healthy subjects (fasting, 7:00–8:00 A.M.)

Population	n	Mean ± SD	Median	Reference range
Men, 20–39 years	1485	95.2 ± 23.2	92	58–146
20–29 years	1159	95.1 ± 22.7	92	57–143
30–39 years	325	95.8 ± 24.9	92	61–164
Men and women, 50–80 years	1138	106.1 ± 28.5	103	55–169
50–59 years	188	105.3 ± 28.3	103	57–167
60–69 years	713	107.3 ± 29.0	105	56–171
70–80 years	237	103.2 ± 27.0	103	55–173
Men, 50–80 years	539	105.2 ± 29.9	102	54–171
Women, 50–80 years	599	106.9 ± 27.2	105	55–166

Reference range of assay: 60–170 U/l.

Table 52. Reference ranges for SGOT (AST; U/l), healthy subjects (fasting, 7:00–8:00 A.M.)

Population	n	Mean ± SD	Median	Reference range
Men, 20–39 years	1334	9.6 ± 3.3	9	6–17
20–29 years	1049	9.7 ± 3.5	9	6–18
30–39 years	285	9.0 ± 2.6	9	6–15
Men and women, 50–80 years	1142	9.2 ± 2.9	9	6–18
50–59 years	190	9.4 ± 3.3	9	5–20
60–69 years	715	9.3 ± 2.8	9	6–18
70–80 years	237	8.9 ± 2.7	8	6–19
Men, 50–80 years	540	9.3 ± 2.9	9	6–17
Women, 50–80 years	602	9.2 ± 2.8	9	5–18

Reference range of assay: men ≤ 18 U/l, women ≤ 15 U/l.

Table 53. Reference ranges for SGPT (ALT; U/l), healthy subjects (fasting, 7:00–8:00 A.M.)

Population	n	Mean ± SD	Median	Reference range
Men, 20–39 years	1333	10.3 ± 5.1	9	5–21
20–29 years	1048	10.3 ± 5.1	9	5–22
30–39 years	285	10.2 ± 5.2	9	5–21
Men and women, 50–80 years	1131	9.5 ± 3.8	9	4–19
50–59 years	189	9.8 ± 3.6	9	5–18
60–69 years	706	9.6 ± 3.9	9	4–19
70–80 years	236	9.1 ± 3.4	8	5–21
Men, 50–80 years	535	9.9 ± 3.7	9	5–19
Women, 50–80 years	596	9.1 ± 3.8	8	4–18

Reference range of assay: men ≤ 22 U/l, women ≤ 17 U/l.

Table 54. Reference ranges for γ-GT (U/l), healthy subjects (fasting, 7:00–8:00 A.M.)

Population	n	Mean ± SD	Median	Reference range
Men, 20–39 years	1333	10.3 ± 4.8	9	5–24
20–29 years	1048	10.3 ± 5.1	9	5–25
30–39 years	285	10.3 ± 3.9	9	6–21
Men and women, 50–80 years	1142	11.3 ± 5.9	10	4–26
50–59 years	190	11.7 ± 6.3	11	5–27
60–69 years	715	11.3 ± 5.8	10	5–26
70–80 years	237	10.8 ± 5.9	9	4–31
Men, 50–80 years	540	13.3 ± 6.2	12	5–29
Women, 50–80 years	602	9.4 ± 4.9	8	4–23

Reference range of assay: men 6–28 U/l, women 4–18 U/l.

Table 55. Reference ranges for LDH (U/l), healthy subjects (fasting, 7:00–8:00 A.M.)

Population	n	Mean ± SD	Median	Reference range
Men, 20–39 years	1346	154.2 ± 43.2	146	97–260
20–29 years	1068	156.0 ± 46.0	147	93–265
30–39 years	278	147.2 ± 28.9	143	106–215
Men and women, 50–80 years	829	173.1 ± 46.5	164	114–303
50–59 years	162	173.6 ± 46.9	162	119–309
60–69 years	516	174.3 ± 47.0	166	116–350
70–80 years	151	168.5 ± 44.3	160	118–380
Men, 50–80 years	423	166.3 ± 48.2	156	112–319
Women, 50–80 years	406	180.2 ± 43.6	173	122–295

Reference range of assay: 140–290 U/l.

Table 56. Reference ranges for total bilirubin (mg/dl), healthy subjects (fasting, 7:00–8:00 A.M.)

Population	n	Mean ± SD	Median	Reference range
Men, 20–39 years	1156	0.51 ± 0.24	0.46	0.20–1.10
20–29 years	923	0.52 ± 0.25	0.48	0.20–1.10
30–39 years	233	0.49 ± 0.21	0.45	0.20–0.91
Men and women, 50–80 years	1095	0.52 ± 0.20	0.48	0.24–1.07
50–59 years	183	0.53 ± 0.20	0.49	0.24–1.05
60–69 years	686	0.53 ± 0.21	0.48	0.23–1.17
70–80 years	226	0.50 ± 0.17	0.48	0.26–1.04
Men, 50–80 years	517	0.56 ± 0.21	0.52	0.25–1.12
Women, 50–80 years	578	0.48 ± 0.19	0.44	0.22–1.03

Reference range of assay: ≤ 1.0 mg/dl.

Table 57. Reference ranges for total bilirubin (μmol/l), healthy subjects (fasting, 7:00–8:00 A.M.)

Population	n	Mean ± SD	Median	Reference range
Men, 20–39 years	1156	8.80 ± 4.17	7.87	3.42–18.81
20–29 years	923	8.90 ± 4.32	8.21	3.42–18.81
30–39 years	233	8.38 ± 3.51	7.70	3.42–15.56
Men and women, 50–80 years	1095	8.89 ± 3.50	8.21	4.10–18.30
50–59 years	183	8.99 ± 3.47	8.38	4.10–17.96
60–69 years	686	8.99 ± 3.66	8.21	3.93–20.01
70–80 years	226	8.49 ± 2.94	8.12	4.45–17.79
Men, 50–80 years	517	9.65 ± 3.55	8.89	4.28–19.16
Women, 50–80 years	578	8.21 ± 3.30	7.53	3.76–17.62

Table 58. Reference ranges for creatinine (mg/dl), healthy subjects (fasting, 7:00–8:00 A.M.)

Population	n	Mean ± SD	Median	Reference range
Men, 20–39 years	1499	0.83 ± 0.12	0.82	0.65–1.11
20–29 years	1171	0.84 ± 0.12	0.82	0.66–1.12
30–39 years	328	0.82 ± 0.11	0.82	0.64–1.09
Men and women, 50–80 years	1095	0.76 ± 0.14	0.75	0.52–1.08
50–59 years	183	0.75 ± 0.14	0.73	0.52–1.06
60–69 years	686	0.76 ± 0.14	0.75	0.52–1.09
70–80 years	226	0.78 ± 0.15	0.78	0.54–1.10
Men, 50–80 years	517	0.84 ± 0.13	0.83	0.61–1.10
Women, 50–80 years	578	0.70 ± 0.12	0.68	0.52–0.98

Reference range of assay: men 0.6–1.1 mg/dl, women 0.5–0.9 mg/dl.

Table 59. Reference ranges for creatinine (µmol/l), healthy subjects (fasting, 7:00–8:00 A.M.)

Population	n	Mean ± SD	Median	Reference range
Men, 20–39 years	1499	73.70 ± 10.54	72.5	57.5–98.1
20–29 years	1171	73.97 ± 10.71	72.5	58.3–99.0
30–39 years	328	72.71 ± 9.89	72.5	56.6–96.4
Men and women, 50–80 years	1095	67.44 ± 12.78	66.3	46.0–95.5
50–59 years	183	66.45 ± 12.41	64.5	46.0–93.7
60–69 years	686	67.35 ± 12.78	66.3	46.0–96.4
70–80 years	226	68.51 ± 13.05	68.5	47.7–97.2
Men, 50–80 years	517	73.96 ± 11.60	73.4	53.9–97.2
Women, 50–80 years	578	61.61 ± 10.82	60.1	46.0–86.6

Table 60. Reference ranges for urea (mg/dl), healthy subjects (fasting, 7:00–8:00 A.M.)

Population	n	Mean ± SD	Median	Reference range
Men, 20–39 years	1177	29.60 ± 8.11	29	16–47
Men and women, 50–80 years	457	33.19 ± 7.98	33	19–51
Men, 50–80 years	226	32.24 ± 7.38	32	19–48
Women, 50–80 years	231	34.13 ± 8.43	33	20–51

Reference range of assay: 10–50 mg/dl.

Table 61. Reference ranges for urea (mmol/l), healthy subjects (fasting, 7:00–8:00 A.M.)

Population	n	Mean ± SD	Median	Reference range
Men, 20–39 years	1177	4.93 ± 1.35	4.8	2.7–7.8
Men and women, 50–80 years	457	5.53 ± 1.33	5.5	3.2–8.5
Men, 50–80 years	226	5.37 ± 1.23	5.3	3.2–8.0
Women, 50–80 years	231	5.68 ± 1.40	5.5	3.3–8.5

Table 62. Reference ranges for uric acid (mg/dl), healthy subjects (fasting, 7:00–8:00 A.M.)

Population	n	Mean ± SD	Median	Reference range
Men 20–39 years	1064	5.33 ± 1.01	5.3	3.4–7.2
20–29 years	774	5.33 ± 1.01	5.3	3.4–7.2
30–39 years	290	5.36 ± 0.92	5.3	3.8–7.3
Men and women, 50–80 years	1092	5.05 ± 1.09	5.0	3.2–7.3
50–59 years	183	5.07 ± 1.00	5.2	3.3–7.1
60–69 years	685	5.04 ± 1.08	5.0	3.2–7.4
70–80 years	224	5.04 ± 1.16	4.9	3.2–8.2
Men 50–80 years	517	5.58 ± 1.05	5.5	3.6–7.8
Women 50–80 years	575	4.57 ± 0.87	4.5	3.0–6.4

Reference range of assay: men 3.4–7.0 mg/dl, women 2.4–5.7 mg/dl.

Table 63. Reference ranges for uric acid (µmol/l), healthy subjects (fasting, 7:00–8:00 A.M.)

Population	n	Mean ± SD	Median	Reference range
Men 20–39 years	1064	316.98 ± 60.35	315.3	202.3–428.3
20–29 years	774	316.98 ± 60.29	315.3	202.3–428.3
30–39 years	290	318.63 ± 54.71	315.3	226.0–434.2
Men and women, 50–80 years	1092	300.20 ± 64.57	297.4	189.8–434.2
50–59 years	183	301.52 ± 59.49	297.4	196.3–422.3
60–69 years	685	300.04 ± 64.36	297.4	190.4–440.2
70–80 years	224	299.60 ± 69.27	291.5	190.4–487.8
Men 50–80 years	517	331.98 ± 62.75	327.2	214.2–464.0
Women 50–80 years	575	271.62 ± 51.54	267.7	178.5–380.7

Table 64. Reference ranges for total cholesterol (mg/dl), healthy subjects (fasting, 7:00–8:00 A.M.)

Population	n	Mean ± SD	Median	Reference range
Men 20–39 years	1449	188.2 ± 34.1	187	124–256
20–29 years	1141	184.6 ± 34.6	183	122–254
30–39 years	308	201.8 ± 28.3	201	152–262
Men and women, 50–80 years	1034	241.9 ± 34.9	243	173–298
50–59 years	174	243.2 ± 35.3	243	172–296
60–69 years	652	242.2 ± 34.7	244	174–298
70–80 years	208	239.7 ± 35.1	238	175–299
Men 50–80 years	517	232.4 ± 35.5	231	171–295
Women 50–80 years	517	251.4 ± 31.6	255	189–299

Reference range of assay: ≤ 200 mg/dl.

Table 65. Reference ranges for total cholesterol (mmol/l), healthy subjects (fasting, 7:00–8:00 A.M.)

Population	n	Mean ± SD	Median	Reference range
Men 20–39 years	1449	4.86 ± 0.88	4.8	3.2–6.6
20–29 years	1141	4.76 ± 0.89	4.7	3.2–6.6
30–39 years	308	5.21 ± 0.73	5.2	3.9–6.8
Men and women, 50–80 years	1034	6.24 ± 0.90	6.3	4.5–7.7
50–59 years	174	6.28 ± 0.91	6.3	4.4–7.6
60–69 years	652	6.25 ± 0.90	6.3	4.5–7.7
70–80 years	208	6.18 ± 0.91	6.1	4.5–7.7
Men 50–80 years	517	6.00 ± 0.92	5.96	4.41–7.61
Women 50–80 years	517	6.48 ± 0.82	6.58	4.88–7.71

Table 66. Reference ranges for triglycerides (mg/dl), healthy subjects (fasting, 7:00–8:00 A.M.)

Population	n	Mean ± SD	Median	Reference range
Men 20–39 years	1105	114.18 ± 57.02	101	45–265
20–29 years	888	115.19 ± 59.38	99	44–276
30–39 years	217	110.03 ± 46.05	103	45–229
Men and women, 50–80 years	994	127.56 ± 53.13	120	56–255
50–59 years	170	137.18 ± 55.99	132	54–257
60–69 years	626	125.59 ± 53.65	112	57–259
70–80 years	198	125.53 ± 48.07	117	60–258
Men 50–80 years	497	135.71 ± 56.19	123	57–260
Women 50–80 years	497	119.41 ± 48.58	110	56–244

Reference range of assay: ≤ 200 mg/dl.

Table 67. Reference ranges for triglycerides (mmol/l), healthy subjects (fasting, 7:00–8:00 A.M.)

Population	n	Mean ± SD	Median	Reference range
Men 20–39 years	1105	1.30 ± 0.65	1.15	0.5–3.0
20–29 years	888	1.31 ± 0.68	1.13	0.5–3.2
30–39 years	217	1.25 ± 0.52	1.17	0.5–2.6
Men and women, 50–80 years	994	1.45 ± 0.61	1.37	0.6–2.9
50–59 years	170	1.56 ± 0.64	1.50	0.6–2.9
60–69 years	626	1.43 ± 0.61	1.28	0.7–3.0
70–80 years	198	1.43 ± 0.55	1.33	0.7–2.9
Men 50–80 years	497	1.55 ± 0.64	1.40	0.7–3.0
Women 50–80 years	497	1.36 ± 0.55	1.25	0.64–2.78

Table 68. Reference ranges for fasting glucose (mg/dl), healthy subjects (fasting, 7:00–8:00 A.M.).

Population	n	Mean ± SD	Median	Reference range
Men 20–39 years	1458	91.3 ± 10.4	91	71–114
20–29 years	1146	90.9 ± 10.7	90	70–114
30–39 years	312	92.7 ± 9.4	92	77–115
Men and women, 50–80 years	1081	100.7 ± 12.6	99	79–129
50–59 years	183	101.5 ± 13.2	99	80–134
60–69 years	675	100.3 ± 12.1	99	79–128
70–80 years	223	101.4 ± 13.5	99	81–135
Men 50–80 years	511	101.8 + 12.3	100	79–133
Women 50–80 years	570	99.7 ± 12.7	98	79–128

Reference range of assay: 76–100 mg/dl.

Table 69. Reference ranges for fasting glucose (mmol/l), healthy subjects (fasting, 7:00–8:00 A.M.)

Population	n	Mean ± SD	Median	Reference range
Men 20–39 years	1458	5.07 ± 0.58	5.1	3.9–6.3
20–29 years	1146	5.05 ± 0.59	5.0	3.9–6.3
30–39 years	312	5.15 ± 0.52	5.1	4.3–6.4
Men and women, 50–80 years	1081	5.59 ± 0.70	5.5	4.4–7.2
50–59 years	183	5.63 ± 0.73	5.5	4.4–7.4
60–69 years	675	5.56 ± 0.67	5.5	4.4–7.1
70–80 years	223	5.62 ± 0.75	5.5	4.5–7.5
Men 50–80 years	511	5.65 ± 0.68	5.6	4.4–7.4
Women 50–80 years	570	5.54 ± 0.70	5.4	4.4–7.1

Table 70. Reference ranges for sodium (mmol/l), healthy subjects (fasting, 7:00–8:00 A.M.)

Population	n	Mean ± SD	Median	Reference range
Men 20–39 years	1375	143.6 ± 2.9	143.7	138.1–149.0
20–29 years	1076	143.7 ± 3.0	143.7	138.1–149.2
30–39 years	299	143.4 ± 2.5	144.0	138.2–147.8
Men and women, 50–80 years	1114	143.1 ± 2.6	143.4	137.3–147.4
50–59 years	179	142.9 ± 2.9	143.4	136.0–147.2
60–69 years	705	143.1 ± 2.5	143.2	137.5–147.6
70–80 years	230	143.4 ± 2.5	143.6	137.8–147.9
Men 50–80 years	524	143.2 ± 2.7	143.5	137.5–147.6
Women 50–80 years	590	143.1 ± 2.5	143.3	137.0–147.0

Reference range of assay: 132–148 mmol/l.

Table 71. Reference ranges for potassium (mmol/l), healthy subjects (fasting, 7:00–8:00 A.M.)

Population	n	Mean ± SD	Median	Reference range
Men 20–39 years	1480	4.36 ± 0.34	4.35	3.73–5.10
20–29 years	1161	4.36 ± 0.34	4.35	3.72–5.10
30–39 years	319	4.39 ± 0.35	4.36	3.80–5.08
Men and women, 50–80 years	1137	4.44 ± 0.36	4.38	3.83–5.30
50–59 years	188	4.44 ± 0.36	4.39	3.80–5.38
60–69 years	712	4.45 ± 0.37	4.40	3.87–5.30
70–80 years	237	4.41 ± 0.35	4.35	3.90–5.26
Men 50–80 years	535	4.45 ± 0.37	4.40	3.79–5.30
Women 50–80 years	602	4.42 ± 0.35	4.37	3.87–5.24

Reference range of assay: 3.6–5.4 mmol/l.

Table 72. Reference ranges for chloride (mmol/l), healthy subjects (fasting, 7:00–8:00 A.M.)

Population	n	Mean ± SD	Median	Reference range
Men 20–39 years	1296	105.8 ± 4.7	105.4	97.8–117.0
20–29 years	1027	106.0 ± 4.9	105.9	97.8–118.0
30–39 years	269	104.9 ± 3.8	105.0	98.1–112.3
Men and women, 50–80 years	952	104.4 ± 3.2	104.4	97.7–110.3
50–59 years	173	104.4 ± 3.2	104.2	97.3–109.9
60–69 years	593	104.4 ± 3.2	104.4	98.0–110.2
70–80 years	186	104.3 ± 3.3	104.3	98.0–110.8
Men 50–80 years	445	104.1 ± 3.3	104.0	97.6–110.5
Women 50–80 years	507	104.6 ± 3.1	104.8	98.0–110.1

Reference range of assay: 94–111 mmol/l.

5.2.6.2 Changes in Clinical Chemistry Parameters After Repeated Measurements

Table 73. Changes in alkaline phosphatase (U/l) after repeated measurements, differences from baseline, healthy subjects (baseline: fasting, 7:00–8:00 A.M.)

Time	n	Mean ± SD	95% diff.[a]	D_{crit}
Men 20–39 years				
24 h	281	0.91 ± 13.69	−25 to 23	21.9
1 week	203	0.59 ± 6.87	−12 to 17	13.2
Men and women, 50–80 years				
24 h	105	−3.47 ± 12.22	−41 to 20	24.0
48 h	127	0.69 ± 6.49	−12 to 13	12.7
1 week	262	1.47 ± 8.16	−15 to 16	15.3
2 weeks	193	1.68 ± 11.28	−23 to 21	21.9

[a] 95% range of differences from baseline.

Table 74. Changes in SGOT (AST; U/l) after repeated measurements, differences from baseline, healthy subjects (baseline: fasting, 7:00–8:00 A.M.)

Time	n	Mean ± SD	95% diff.[a]	D_{crit}
Men 20–39 years				
24 h	261	0.27 ± 2.69	–4 to 6	4.3
1 week	203	0.00 ± 1.56	–2 to 3	3.0
Men and women, 50–80 years				
24 h	125	0.39 ± 2.87	–5 to 9	5.6
48 h	131	–0.42 ± 2.41	–5 to 4	4.4
1 week	263	–0.22 ± 2.25	–5 to 4	4.7
2 weeks	215	–0.18 ± 2.84	–8 to 5	5.3

[a] 95% range of differences from baseline.

Table 75. Changes in SGPT (ALT; U/l) after repeated measurements, differences from baseline, healthy subjects (baseline: fasting, 7:00–8:00 A.M.)

Time	n	Mean ± SD	95% diff.[a]	D_{crit}
Men 20–39 years				
24 h	261	0.62 ± 3.27	–5 to 7	5.3
1 week	203	0.29 ± 1.95	–3 to 5	3.6
Men and women, 50–80 years				
24 h	125	–0.16 ± 2.03	–4 to 6	4.0
48 h	141	0.07 ± 1.70	–3 to 3	3.3
1 week	259	–0.06 ± 2.08	–5 to 3	3.6
2 weeks	215	–0.37 ± 2.85	–9 to 4	5.5

[a] 95% range of differences from baseline.

Table 76. Changes in γ-GT (U/l) after repeated measurements, differences from baseline, healthy subjects (baseline: fasting, 7:00–8:00 A.M.)

Time	n	Mean ± SD	95% diff.[a]	D_{crit}
Men 20–39 years				
24 h	261	0.82 ± 1.66	–1 to 5	3.3
1 week	203	–0.89 ± 1.27	–4 to 2	2.4
Men and women, 50–80 years				
24 h	125	–0.24 ± 1.39	–3 to 3	2.7
48 h	141	–0.11 ± 1.39	–3 to 2	2.7
1 week	263	–0.07 ± 1.84	–4 to 4	4.1
2 weeks	195	–0.15 ± 2.86	–6 to 5	5.6

[a] 95% range of differences from baseline.

Table 77. Changes in LDH (U/l) after repeated measurements, differences from baseline, healthy subjects (baseline: fasting, 7:00–8:00 A.M.)

Time	n	Mean ± SD	95% diff.[a]	D_{crit}
Men 20–39 years				
24 h	257	−1.98 ± 38.09	−93 to 87	56.9
1 week	199	0.46 ± 17.29	−46 to 39	33.2
Men and women, 50–80 years				
24 h	79	1.01 ± 19.72	−39 to 40	38.5
48 h	123	−4.58 ± 20.91	−52 to 31	40.0
1 week	213	−2.69 ± 23.40	−61 to 46	48.7
2 weeks	171	−1.33 ± 36.98	−86 to 77	67.6

[a] 95% range of differences from baseline.

Table 78. Changes in total bilirubin (mg/dl) after repeated measurements, differences from baseline, healthy subjects (baseline: fasting, 7:00–8:00 A.M.)

Time	n	Mean ± SD	95% diff.[a]	D_{crit}
Men 20–39 years				
24 h	254	0.01 ± 0.38	−0.7 to 0.7	0.7
1 week	202	0.01 ± 0.34	−0.1 to 0.1	0.1
Men and women, 50–80 years				
24 h	125	−0.03 ± 0.13	−0.3 to 0.2	0.2
48 h	141	−0.02 ± 0.14	−0.3 to 0.3	0.3
1 week	263	0.00 ± 0.15	−0.3 to 0.3	0.3
2 weeks	215	0.00 ± 0.17	−0.3 to 0.4	0.3

[a] 95% range of differences from baseline.

Table 79. Changes in total bilirubin (μmol/l) after repeated measurements, differences from baseline, healthy subjects (baseline: fasting, 7:00–8:00 A.M.)

Time	n	Mean ± SD	95% diff.[a]	D_{crit}
Men 20–39 years				
24 h	254	0.24 ± 6.43	−11.6 to 11.9	11.4
1 week	202	0.26 ± 5.75	−1.4 to 2.2	2.1
Men and women, 50–80 years				
24 h	125	−0.54 ± 2.17	−4.6 to 3.8	4.0
48 h	141	−0.40 ± 2.48	−5.6 to 4.3	4.3
1 week	263	−0.06 ± 2.51	−5.1 to 4.8	4.6
2 weeks	215	−0.05 ± 2.94	−5.8 to 6.0	5.4

[a] 95% range of differences from baseline.

Table 80. Changes in creatinine (mg/dl) after repeated measurements, differences from baseline, healthy subjects (baseline: fasting, 7:00–8:00 A.M.)

Time	n	Mean ± SD	95% diff.[a]	D_{crit}
Men 20–39 years				
24 h	284	0.01 ± 0.13	−0.26 to 0.30	0.24
1 week	203	0.00 ± 0.07	−0.14 to 0.17	0.13
Men and women, 50–80 years				
24 h	105	0.00 ± 0.05	−0.11 to 0.11	0.10
48 h	113	−0.01 ± 0.05	−0.10 to 0.09	0.09
1 week	263	0.01 ± 0.08	−0.15 to 0.16	0.15
2 weeks	215	0.01 ± 0.09	−0.18 to 0.19	0.16

[a] 95% range of differences from baseline.

Table 81. Changes in creatinine (µmol/l) after repeated measurements, differences from baseline, healthy subjects (baseline: fasting, 7:00–8:00 A.M.)

Time	n	Mean ± SD	95% diff.[a]	D_{crit}
Men 20–39 years				
24 h	284	0.45 ± 11.69	−23.0 to 26.5	21.0
1 week	203	−0.05 ± 6.03	−12.4 to 15.0	11.9
Men and women, 50–80 years				
24 h	105	−0.05 ± 4.57	−9.7 to 9.7	8.8
48 h	113	−1.02 ± 4.23	−8.8 to 8.0	8.1
1 week	263	0.49 ± 6.85	−13.3 to 14.1	13.3
2 weeks	215	0.50 ± 7.56	−15.9 to 16.8	14.1

[a] 95% range of differences from baseline.

Table 82. Changes in uric acid (mg/dl) after repeated measurements, differences from baseline, healthy subjects (baseline: fasting, 7:00–8:00 A.M.)

Time	n	Mean ± SD	95% diff.[a]	D_{crit}
Men 20–39 years				
24 h	189	−0.14 ± 0.77	−1.7 to 1.4	1.5
1 week	145	0.03 ± 0.63	−1.0 to 1.2	1.2
Men and women, 50–80 years				
24 h	125	−0.01 ± 0.48	−0.9 to 1.0	0.9
48 h	141	−0.05 ± 0.56	−1.2 to 0.9	1.1
1 week	263	0.10 ± 0.63	−1.1 to 1.4	1.3
2 weeks	215	0.14 ± 0.64	−1.1 to 1.5	1.2

[a] 95% range of differences from baseline.

Table 83. Changes in uric acid (µmol/l) after repeated measurements, differences from baseline, healthy subjects (baseline: fasting, 7:00–8:00 A.M.)

Time	n	Mean ± SD	95% diff.[a]	D_{crit}
Men 20–39 years				
24 h	189	–8.09 ± 45.59	–101.1 to 83.3	90.3
1 week	145	1.81 ± 37.45	–59.5 to 71.4	73.1
Men and women, 50–80 years				
24 h	125	–0.67 ± 28.67	–53.5 to 59.5	54.1
48 h	141	–3.12 ± 33.56	–71.4 to 53.5	65.9
1 week	263	5.77 ± 37.36	–65.4 to 83.3	78.5
2 weeks	215	8.33 ± 38.31	–65.4 to 89.2	71.9

[a] 95% range of differences from baseline.

Table 84. Changes in total cholesterol (mg/dl) after repeated measurements, differences from baseline, healthy subjects (baseline: fasting, 7:00–8:00 A.M.)

Time	n	Mean ± SD	95% diff.[a]	D_{crit}
Men 20–39 years				
24 h	279	2.47 ± 18.39	–34 to 38	33.9
1 week	203	–0.15 ± 10.14	–22 to 20	19.7
Men and women, 50–80 years				
24 h	115	3.02 ± 13.57	–19 to 29	26.4
48 h	141	–1.10 ± 13.49	–29 to 25	26.1
1 week	233	0.78 ± 16.90	–29 to 34	32.7
2 weeks	205	0.46 ± 20.11	–37 to 36	38.7

[a] 95% range of differences from baseline.

Table 85. Changes in total cholesterol (mmol/l) after repeated measurements, differences from baseline, healthy subjects (baseline: fasting, 7:00–8:00 A.M.)

Time	n	Mean ± SD	95% diff.[a]	D_{crit}
Men 20–39 years				
24 h	279	0.06 ± 0.47	–0.9 to 1.0	0.9
1 week	203	0.00 ± 0.26	–0.6 to 0.5	0.5
Men and women, 50–80 years				
24 h	115	0.08 ± 0.35	–0.5 to 0.8	0.7
48 h	141	–0.03 ± 0.35	–0.8 to 0.7	0.7
1 week	233	0.02 ± 0.44	–0.8 to 0.9	0.8
2 weeks	205	0.01 ± 0.52	–1.0 to 0.9	1.0

[a] 95% range of differences from baseline.

Table 86. Changes in fasting glucose (mg/dl) after repeated measurements, differences from baseline, healthy subjects (baseline: fasting, 7:00–8:00 A.M.)

Time	n	Mean ± SD	95% diff.[a]	D_{crit}
Men 20–39 years				
24 h	282	−0.99 ± 11.55	−24 to 25	19.2
1 week	203	0.79 ± 5.80	−10 to 12	11.0
Men and women, 50–80 years				
24 h	125	−0.15 ± 13.70	−23 to 19	23.9
48 h	141	−1.33 ± 7.82	−16 to 12	14.8
1 week	256	0.79 ± 8.86	−17 to 18	16.3
2 weeks	214	0.35 ± 10.80	−20 to 23	18.9

[a] 95% range of differences from baseline.

Table 87. Changes in fasting glucose (mmol/l) after repeated measurements, differences from baseline, healthy subjects (baseline: fasting, 7:00–8:00 A.M.)

Time	n	Mean ± SD	95% diff.[a]	D_{crit}
Men 20–39 years				
24 h	282	−0.06 ± 0.64	−1.3 to 1.4	1.1
1 week	203	0.04 ± 0.32	−0.6 to 0.7	0.6
Men and women, 50–80 years				
24 h	125	−0.01 ± 0.76	−1.3 to 1.1	1.3
48 h	141	−0.07 ± 0.43	−0.9 to 0.7	0.8
1 week	256	0.04 ± 0.49	−0.9 to 1.0	0.9
2 weeks	214	0.02 ± 0.60	−1.1 to 1.3	1.1

[a] 95% range of differences from baseline.

Table 88. Changes in sodium (mmol/l) after repeated measurements, differences from baseline, healthy subjects (baseline: fasting, 7:00–8:00 A.M.)

Time	n	Mean ± SD	95% diff.[a]	D_{crit}
Men 20–39 years				
24 h	281	0.02 ± 1.39	−2.7 to 1.8	1.9
1 week	203	0.00 ± 0.71	−1.1 to 1.4	1.2
Men and women, 50–80 years				
24 h	125	0.12 ± 2.10	−3.1 to 3.7	4.0
48 h	141	0.20 ± 2.22	−4.3 to 4.5	4.3
1 week	263	0.01 ± 1.00	−1.8 to 1.7	1.7
2 weeks	203	0.14 ± 1.81	−3.2 to 2.8	3.4

[a] 95% range of differences from baseline.

Table 89. Changes in potassium (mmol/l) after repeated measurements, differences from baseline, healthy subjects (baseline: fasting, 7:00–8:00 A.M.)

Time	n	Mean ± SD	95% diff.[a]	D_{crit}
Men 20–39 years				
24 h	203	−0.03 ± 0.39	−0.7 to 0.9	0.7
1 week	203	−0.02 ± 0.33	−0.7 to 0.6	0.6
Men and women, 50–80 years				
24 h	125	0.20 ± 0.50	−0.7 to 0.9	0.8
48 h	141	0.02 ± 0.39	−0.8 to 0.9	0.8
1 week	263	−0.01 ± 0.28	−0.6 to 0.6	0.5
2 weeks	215	0.09 ± 0.44	−0.9 to 0.9	0.8

[a] 95% range of differences from baseline.

5.2.6.3 Confirmatory Statistics of Clinical Chemistry Parameters

Baseline Values

Table 90. Comparison of differences in clinical chemistry parameters between selected subject groups: statistical significance

	Elderly vs. young	Elderly men vs. young men	Elderly men vs. elderly women	50–59 years vs. 60–69 years	50–59 years vs. 70–80 years	60–69 years vs. 70–80 years	20–29 years vs. 50–59 years	20–29 years vs. 30–39 years
Alkaline phosphatase	–	–	ns	ns	ns	ns	–	–
AST (SGOT)	++	+	ns	ns	+	++	ns	++
ALT (SGPT)	++	ns	++	ns	+	ns	++	++
γ-GT	++	++	++	ns	+	ns	++	++
LDH	++	++	++	ns	ns	ns	++	++
Total bilirubin	+	++	++	ns	ns	ns	++	++
Creatinine	++	ns	++	ns	ns	ns	ns	++
Blood urea (BUN)	++	++	+	+	++	ns	ns	ns
Uric acid	++	++	++	ns	ns	ns	ns	ns
Total protein	+	ns	+	ns	ns	ns	++	++
Total cholesterol	++	++	++	ns	ns	ns	++	++
Triglycerides	++	++	++	+	ns	ns	++	++
Glucose fasting	++	++	++	ns	ns	ns	++	++
Calcium	ns	ns	ns	++	ns	ns	(+)	ns
Sodium	++	+	ns	ns	++	+	ns	++
Potassium	++	++	ns	ns	ns	ns	++	++
Chlorine	++	++	++	ns	ns	ns	ns	++

++, $p \leq 0.01$; +, $p \leq 0.05$; ns, not significant (two-tailed p values, Mann–Whitney U–Wilcoxon rank sum W test);
– no values in young subjects.

5.2.6.3.2 Repeated Measurements

Table 91. Comparison of clinical chemistry parameters after repeated measurements: statistical significance

	24 h	48 h	1 week	2 weeks	3 weeks
Elderly					
Alkaline phosphatase	++	ns	++	++	ns
AST (SGOT)	ns	ns	ns	ns	ns
ALT (SGPT)	ns	ns	ns	ns	ns
γ-GT	ns	ns	ns	ns	ns
LDH	ns	+	ns	ns	ns
Total bilirubin	++	ns	ns	ns	ns
Creatinine	ns	+	ns	ns	ns
Uric acid	ns	ns	+	++	+
Total protein	ns	ns	ns	ns	ns
Total cholesterol	+	ns	ns	ns	ns
Triglycerides	ns	ns	ns	ns	ns
Glucose fasting	ns	ns	ns	ns	ns
Sodium	ns	ns	ns	ns	++
Potassium	++	ns	ns	++	ns
Chlorine	+	++	+	ns	ns
Young					
Alkaline phosphatase	ns	–	ns	–	–
AST (SGOT)	ns	–	ns	–	–
ALT (SGPT)	++	–	ns	–	–
γ-GT	++	–	++	–	–
LDH	ns	–	ns	–	–
Creatinine	ns	–	ns	–	–
Blood urea (BUN)	+	–	+	–	–
Uric acid	+	–	ns	–	–
Total protein	ns	–	ns	–	–
Total cholesterol	ns	–	ns	–	–
Glucose fasting	ns	–	ns	–	–

++, $p \leq 0.01$; +, $p \leq 0.05$; *ns*, not significant; – no values (versus baseline, two-tailed p values, Wilcoxon matched-pairs signed-rank test).

5.2.7 Hematology

5.2.7.1 Baseline Values

Table 92. Reference ranges for leukocytes (10^9/l), healthy subjects (fasting, 7:00–9:00 A.M.)

Population	n	Mean ± SD	Median	Reference range
Men 20–39 years	1434	6.47 ± 1.63	6.2	4.3–10.7
20–29 years	1123	6.39 ± 1.54	6.1	4.3–10.6
30–39 years	311	6.78 ± 1.91	6.5	4.3–11.5
Men and women, 50–80 years	1102	6.49 ± 1.45	6.1	4.8–10.4
50–59 years	322	6.53 ± 1.60	6.1	4.7–10.9
60–69 years	603	6.54 ± 1.46	6.1	4.8–10.4
70–80 years	177	6.26 ± 1.09	6.0	5.0–9.4
Men 50–80 years	489	6.68 ± 1.61	6.1	4.9–10.9
Women 50–80 years	613	6.35 ± 1.30	6.0	4.8 –10.1

Reference range: 4.3–10 10^9/l.

Table 93. Reference ranges for erythrocytes (10^{12}/l), healthy subjects (fasting, 7:00–9:00 A.M.)

Population	n	Mean ± SD	Median	Reference range
Men 20–39 years	1445	4.91± 0.36	4.89	4.28–5.60
20–29 years	1138	4.92 ± 0.36	4.91	4.28 –5.60
30–39 years	307	4.86 ± 0.36	4.84	4.33–5.58
Men and women, 50–80 years	1102	4.60 ± 0.37	4.61	3.94–5.32
50–59 years	322	4.58 ± 0.33	4.60	3.92–5.22
60–69 years	603	4.63 ± 0.39	4.62	3.94–5.41
70–80 years	177	4.55 ± 0.37	4.60	3.90–5.30
Men 50–80 years	489	4.81 ± 0.30	4.80	4.19–5.40
Women 50–80 years	613	4.44 ± 0.33	4.40	3.89–5.14

Reference range: 4.4–6.0 10^{12}/l.

Table 94. Reference ranges for hemoglobin (g/dl), healthy subjects (fasting, 7:00–9:00 A.M.)

Population	n	Mean ± SD	Median	Reference range
Men 20–39 years	1482	14.87 ± 1.04	14.9	12.8–16.9
20–29 years	1156	14.92 ± 1.02	15.0	12.8–16.8
30–39 years	326	14.72 ± 1.09	14.7	12.7–17.1
Men and women, 50–80 years	1102	13.91 ± 1.30	13.9	11.4–16.3
50–59 years	322	13.79 ± 1.16	13.7	11.7–16.0
60–69 years	603	14.03 ± 1.37	14.1	11.3–16.4
70–80 years	177	13.71 ± 1.24	13.7	11.4–16.2
Men 50–80 years	489	14.80 ± 0.99	14.8	13.2–13.5
Women 50–80 years	613	13.20 ± 1.04	13.2	11.2–15.4

Reference range: men 14–18 g/dl, women 12–16 g/dl.

Table 95. Reference ranges for hematocrit (%), healthy subjects (fasting, 7:00–9:00 A.M.)

Population	n	Mean ± SD	Median	Reference range
Men 20–39 years	1492	43.98 ± 3.33	44.0	37.6–50.4
20–29 years	1164	44.12 ± 3.30	44.2	37.6–50.5
30–39 years	328	43.48 ± 3.41	43.5	37.0–49.9
Men and women, 50–80 years	969	41.86 ± 3.62	41.8	34.4–49.0
50–59 years	249	41.68 ± 2.99	41.4	36.6–47.6
60–69 years	547	42.26 ± 3.77	42.4	34.3–49.4
70–80 years	173	40.84 ± 3.72	40.2	34.4–48.7
Men 50–80 years	489	43.82 ± 3.01	44.1	38.6–49.4
Women 50–80 years	480	39.86 ± 3.04	39.7	34.0–45.9

Reference range: 37%–52%

Table 96. Reference ranges for platelets (10^9/l), healthy subjects (fasting, 7:00–9:00 A.M.)

Population	n	Mean ± SD	Median	Reference range
Men 20–39 years	1415	239.73 ± 45.08	234	170–343
20–29 years	1104	239.58 ± 45.54	235	170–342
30–39 years	311	240.25 ± 43.51	233	176–352
Men and women, 50–80 years	1100	248.19 ± 60.15	239	156–405
50–59 years	322	239.95 ± 46.70	240	161–341
60–69 years	602	252.07 ± 62.66	241	155–325
70–80 years	176	250.01 ± 71.11	230	153–467
Men 50–80 years	487	233.34 ± 53.16	228	152–364
Women 50–80 years	613	259.99 ± 62.76	246	173–418

Reference range: men 130–400 10^9/l, women 130–300 10^9/l.

Table 97. Reference ranges for lymphocytes (% of differential count), healthy subjects (fasting, 7:00–9:00 A.M.)

Population	n	Mean ± SD	Median	Reference range
Men 20–39 years	1397	38.26 ± 7.94	38	25–55
20–29 years	1090	38.44 ± 7.85	38	25–55
30–39 years	307	37.62 ± 8.22	36	25–55
Men and women, 50–80 years	1090	33.58 ± 7.81	33	20–49
50–59 years	316	34.46 ± 7.73	34	21–49
60–69 years	600	32.87 ± 7.76	32	20–49
70–80 years	174	34.41 ± 7.96	34	19–54
Men 50–80 years	483	32.33 ± 7.63	32	19–49
Women 50–80 years	607	34.57 ± 7.82	34	21–50

Reference range: 20.5–51.1% of differential count

Table 98. Reference ranges for segmented neutrophils (% of differential count), healthy subjects (fasting, 7:00–9:00 A.M.)

Population	n	Mean ± SD	Median	Reference range
Men 20–39 years	1087	55.09 ± 8.36	55	39–72
20–29 years	865	55.17 ± 8.47	55	39–72
30–39 years	222	54.77 ± 7.93	55	40–69
Men and women, 50–80 years	1089	59.60 ± 8.13	60	44–75
50–59 years	316	59.59 ± 8.27	59	45–76
60–69 years	599	60.01 ± 8.01	61	44–74
70–80 years	174	58.20 ± 8.19	58	44–85
Men 50–80 years	483	59.90 ± 7.87	60	45–75
Women 50–80 years	606	59.36 ± 8.34	60	44–75

Reference range: 41.2%–70.1%

Table 99. Reference ranges for Quick's test (%), healthy subjects (fasting, 7:00–9:00 A.M.)

Population	n	Mean ± SD	Median	Reference range
Men 20–39 years	1387	104.65 ± 12.00	104	82–130
20–29 years	1100	104.50 ± 12.17	104	82–130
30–39 years	287	105.26 ± 11.29	105	82–132
Men and women, 50–80 years	953	113.54 ± 11.75	113	93–138
50–59 years	246	114.78 ± 11.40	114	95–146
60–69 years	537	113.36 ± 12.22	113	91–138
70–80 years	170	112.31 ± 10.60	111	92–139
Men 50–80 years	480	112.80 ± 12.06	112	90–138
Women 50–80 years	473	114.29 ± 11.39	113	94–138

Reference range: 70–130%

5.2.7.2 Changes After Repeated Measurements

Table 100. Changes in leukocytes (10^9/l) after repeated measurements, differences from baseline, healthy subjects (baseline: fasting, 7:00–8:00 A.M.)

Time	n	Mean ± SD	95% diff.[a]	D_{crit}
Men and women 50–80 years				
24 h	211	–0.02 ± 0.98	–2.2 to 2.1	2.1
1 week	240	–0.02 ± 0.89	–1.9 to 1.9	1.8
2 weeks	225	–0.16 ± 0.82	–1.7 to 1.5	1.8
3 weeks	172	–0.26 ± 0.85	–1.7 to 1.6	1.6

[a] 95% range of differences from baseline.

Table 101. Changes in erythrocytes (10^{12}/l) after repeated measurements, differences from baseline, healthy subjects (baseline: fasting, 7:00–8:00 A.M.)

Time	n	Mean ± SD	95% diff.[a]	D_{crit}
Men and women, 50–80 years				
24 h	211	−0.09 ± 0.24	−0.63 to 0.40	0.5
1 week	240	−0.02 ± 0.20	−0.42 to 0.32	0.4
2 weeks	225	−0.06 ± 0.22	−0.53 to 0.33	0.4
3 weeks	172	−0.06 ± 0.24	−0.60 to 0.54	0.5

[a] 95% range of differences from baseline.

Table 102. Changes in hemoglobin (g/dl) after repeated measurements, differences from baseline, healthy subjects (baseline: fasting, 7:00–8:00 A.M.)

Time	n	Mean ± SD	95% diff.[a]	D_{crit}
Men and women, 50–80 years				
24 h	211	−0.33 ± 0.80	−2.5 to 1.0	1.6
1 week	240	−0.10 ± 0.57	−1.2 to 1.1	1.1
2 weeks	225	−0.22 ± 0.62	−1.5 to 1.0	1.2
3 weeks	172	−0.22 ± 0.59	−1.3 to 1.3	1.2

[a] 95% range of differences from baseline.

Table 103. Changes in hematocrit (%) after repeated measurements, differences from baseline, healthy subjects (baseline: fasting, 7:00–8:00 A.M.)

Time	n	Mean ± SD	95% diff.[a]	D_{crit}
Men and women, 50–80 years				
24 h	211	−0.89 ± 2.10	−6.0 to 3.2	4.1
1 week	240	−0.44 ± 2.07	−4.4 to 3.3	4.0
2 weeks	225	−0.60 ± 2.14	−4.6 to 2.8	4.1
3 weeks	172	−0.74 ± 2.92	−6.9 to 5.8	5.6

[a] 95% range of differences from baseline.

Table 104. Changes in platelets (10^9/l) after repeated measurements, differences from baseline, healthy subjects (baseline: fasting, 7:00–8:00 A.M.)

Time	n	Mean ± SD	95% diff.[a]	D_{crit}
Men and women, 50–80 years				
24 h	211	−2.68 ± 27.61	−83 to 56	53.7
1 week	240	4.35 ± 20.96	−37 to 48	40.7
2 weeks	225	5.28 ± 18.69	−31 to 39	45.2
3 weeks	172	1.53 ± 24.13	−44 to 50	46.3

[a] 95% range of differences from baseline.

Table 105. Changes in lymphocytes (%) after repeated measurements, differences from baseline, , healthy subjects (baseline: fasting, 7:00–8:00 A.M.)

Time	n	Mean ± SD	95% diff.[a]	D_{crit}
Men and women, 50–80 years				
24 h	200	0.97 ± 5.74	−10 to 12	11.1
1 week	218	−0.22 ± 5.66	−13 to 10	10.3
2 weeks	199	−1.09 ± 6.17	−14 to 11	12.4
3 weeks	172	−0.57 ± 8.46	−17 to 17	16.0

[a] 95% range of differences from baseline.

Table 106. Changes in segmented neutrophils (%) after repeated measurements, differences from baseline, healthy subjects (baseline: fasting, 7:00–8:00 A.M.)

Time	n	Mean ± SD	95% diff.[a]	D_{crit}
Men and women, 50–80 years				
24 h	211	−0.88 ± 7.15	−15 to 17	8.2
1 week	179	0.03 ± 0.47	−1 to 1	0.8
2 weeks	195	0.02 ± 0.39	−1 to 1	0.7
3 weeks	162	0.07 ± 0.59	−1 to 1	0.5

[a] 95% range of differences from baseline.

Table 107. Changes in Quick's test (%) after repeated measurements, differences from baseline, healthy subjects (baseline: fasting, 7:00–8:00 A.M.)

Time	n	Mean ± SD	95% diff.[a]	D_{crit}
Men and women, 50–80 years				
24 h	200	−0.27 ± 7.20	−12 to 12	13.2
1 week	230	0.94 ± 8.05	−14 to 16	15.3
2 weeks	211	1.37 ± 8.08	−15 to 17	14.6
3 weeks	162	1.10 ± 9.97	−18 to 24	19.4

[a] 95% range of differences from baseline.

5.2.7.3 Confirmatory Statistics of Hematological Parameters

Baseline Values

Table 108. Comparison of hematological parameters between selected subject groups

	Elderly men vs. young men	Elderly men vs. elderly women	50–59 years vs. 60–69 years	50–59 years vs. 70–80 years	60–69 years vs. 70–80 years	20–29 years vs. 50–59 years, men	20–29 years vs. 30–39 years
Leukocytes	ns	++	ns	ns	ns	++	++
Erythrocytes	++	++	ns	ns	+	++	++
Hemoglobin	ns	++	++	ns	++	++	++
Hematocrit	ns	++	+	++	++	++	++
MCV	++	++	++	ns	ns	ns	++
MCHC	ns	++	++	ns	ns	ns	ns
Platelets	++	++	+	ns	ns	ns	ns
Lymphocytes	++	++	++	ns	+	++	+
Monocytes	+	++	++	++	ns	ns	++
Eosinophils	ns	++	ns	ns	ns	ns	++
Basophils	ns	ns	ns	ns	ns	ns	ns
Segm. neutrophils	++	ns	ns	ns	++	++	ns
Bands	ns	ns	ns	ns	ns	ns	ns
Quick's test	++	ns	ns	+	ns	++	ns

++, $p \leq 0.01$; +, $p \leq 0.05$; *ns*, not significant (two-tailed p values, Mann–Whitney U–Wilcoxon rank sum W test. *MCV*, mean corpuscular volume; *MCHC*, mean corpuscular hemoglobin concentration.

Repeated Measurements

Table 109. Hematological parameters on different study days, comparison with baseline, men and women aged 50–80 years: statistical significance

	24 h	1 week	2 weeks	3 weeks
Leukocytes	ns	ns	ns	++
Erythrocytes	++	+	++	++
Hemoglobin	++	++	++	++
Hematocrit	++	++	++	++
MCV	ns	++	++	++
MCH	ns	ns	ns	+
MCHC	+	ns	ns	ns
Platelets	ns	++	++	ns
Lymphocytes	+	ns	ns	ns
Monocytes	+	ns	ns	ns
Eosinophils	ns	ns	ns	ns
Basophils	ns	ns	ns	ns
Seg neutros	+	ns	ns	ns
Reticulocytes	++	++	++	++
Bands	ns	ns	ns	ns
Quick's test	ns	ns	ns	ns

++, $p \leq 0.01$; +, $p \leq 0.05$; *ns*, not significant (versus baseline, two-tailed p values, Wilcoxon matched-pairs signed-rank test).

MCV, mean corpuscular volume; *MCH*, mean corpuscular hemoglobin; *MCHC*, mean corpuscular hemoglobin concentration.

5.2.8 Adverse Events

Signs, Symptoms. Among 253 inhouse subjects under placebo aged 50–80 years, 42 reported the symptoms listed in Table 110 (without consideration of repeated nominations; some subjects reported several symptoms).

Objective Findings. Four of the 253 placebo subjects developed hypertension with diastolic blood pressure values $\geq$ 105 mmHg. Eight subjects developed ECG changes: AV block of second degree, two subjects; ST depression, three subjects ; ventricular arrhythmias, two subjects; and supraventicular arrhythmia, one subject. One subject developed silent myocardial infarction, and four rush or urticarialike dermatological symptoms.

Laboratory Findings. Eight of the 253 subjects with normal baseline values had transaminases above the double upper reference range. One subject developed thrombocytopenia (72 000 thrombocytes).

5.3 Consequences from Experimental Data in Healthy Subjects

The present data from healthy elderly participants in clinical pharmacology studies closely match those from elderly patients reported in the literature; they

Table 110. Adverse events, healthy subjects aged 50–80 years (42/253)

Symptom	Number with adverse events	Number with mild intensity	Number with moderate intensity	Number with severe intensity
Headache	8	5	4	—
Tiredness	5	3	2	1
Dizziness	4	3	1	—
Back pain	3	2	1	—
Drowsiness	3	3	—	—
Peripheral paresthesia	2	1	1	—
Attacks of weakness	2	2	—	—
Inner restlessnee	2	1	1	—
Dry mouth	2	1	1	—
Nausea	2	2	—	—
Sleepiness	2	1	1	—
Arthralgia	3	2	1	—
Pressure in heart region	3	3	—	—
Blurred vision	1		1	—
Rheumatic pain	3	1	1	1
Inspiratory difficulties	1	1	—	—

clearly indicate that many — but not all — variables change with age. The majority of these changes can already be demonstrated in the group of 50–59 year-olds, a finding which is also in agreement with individual observations in the literature.

Large differences are demonstrable in the upper (but not the lower) limits of supine and standing systolic and diastolic blood pressures (Table 111). In

Table 111. Reference ranges, coefficient of variation, and Dcrit of blood pressure and pulse rate, young and elderly subjects

	Reference range	CV (%)	D_{crit} 1 week
Supine			
Systolic BP (mmHg)			
Men and women, 50–80 years	100–162	13.45	13.6
Men, 20–39 years	100–142	8.79	8.9
Diastolic BP (mmHg)			
Men and women, 50–80 years	64–98	12.08	11.5
Men, 20–39 years	60–90	10.37	9.6
Pulse rate (bpm)			
Men and women, 50–80 years	52–87	13.24	18.1
Men, 20–39 years	50–84	13.43	11.3
Standing			
Systolic BP (mmHg)			
Men and women, 50–80 years	98–168	13.75	—
Men, 20–39 years	100–142	9.12	—
Diastolic BP (mmHg)			
Men and women, 50–80 years	62–102	12.33	—
Men, 20–39 years	62–98	10.77	—
Pulse rate (bpm)			
Men and women, 50–80 years	59–98	13.38	—
Men, 20–39 years	60–100	13.36	—

contrast, the typical decrease in pulse rate with age described in the past by several groups cannot be detected in the reported population of healthy elderly subjects. Moreover, ECG times (Table 112) are in fact not influenced by age.

Table 112. Reference ranges and coefficient of variation of ECG of times, young and elderly subjects

	Reference range	CV (%)
RR (s)		
Men and women, 50–80 years	0.69–1.19	13.90
Men, 20–39 years	0.73–1.30	14.93
P (s)		
Men and women, 50–80 years	0.08–0.13	13.28
Men, 20–39 years	0.08–0.12	11.71
PQ (s)		
Men and women, 50–80 years	0.12–0.20	12.89
Men, 20–39 years	0.12–0.20	13.10
QRS (s)		
Men and women, 50–80 years	0.07–0.11	11.56
Men, 20–39 years	0.07–0.11	11.81
QT (s)		
Men and women, 50–80 years	0.35–0.44	6.32
Men, 20–39 years	0.33–0.43	6.99
QTC (s)		
Men and women, 50–80 years	0.37–0.44	4.53
Men, 20–39 years	0.34–0.43	6.04
Heart rate (bpm)		
Men and women, 50–80 years	50–87	14.36
Men, 20–39 years	46–82	15.57

While several clinical chemistry parameters (cholesterol, triglycerides, glucose, alkaline phosphatase) and hematological parameters (erythrocytes, hemoglobin) differ significantly between young and elderly subjects, others do not (Tables 113, 114) and show means that are practically identical in both groups or differ only marginally. Values determined from women are often significantly different from those of men; indeed the effect of sex seems in many parameters to be more relevant than that of age.

The intersubject variation of reference ranges (expressed as coefficient of variation) is in most cases similar in young and elderly subjects. It therefore cannot be concluded from the present data that the reference ranges for elderly subjects are wider than for the young population, as has been described previously for elderly patients.

The important question which arises from these findings in healthy subjects is whether it is necessary to use special sets of stratified reference ranges for elderly people. For clinical and therapeutic purposes, specific reference ranges in elderly persons are probably not necessary. The situation is different, however, in clinical pharmacology, where even minor changes or deviations from the "norm," that are often not at all relevant for diagnostic procedures, can be important for inclusion of truly healthy study participants, for the calculation of sample size and especially for an interpretation of study results. While it is

Table 113. Reference ranges, coefficient of variation, and Dcrit of clinical chemistry variables, young and elderly subjects

	Reference range	CV (%)	D_{crit} 1 week
Alkaline phosphatase (U/l)			
Men and women, 50–80 years	55–169	26.85	15.3
Men, 20–39 years	58–146	24.38	13.2
AST (SGOT; U/l)			
Men and women, 50–80 years	6–18	31.11	4.7
Men, 20–39 years	6–17	34.69	3.0
ALT (SGPT; U/l)			
Men and women, 50–80 years	4–19	39.46	3.6
Men, 20–39 years	5–21	49.82	3.6
γ-GT (U/l)			
Men and women, 50–80 years	4–26	52.11	4.1
Men, 20–39 years	5–24	47.14	2.4
LDH (U/l)			
Men and women, 50–80 years	114–303	26.84	48.7
Men, 20–39 years	97–260	28.01	33.2
Total bilirubin (mg/dl)			
Men and women, 50–80 years	0.24–1.07	39.35	0.27
Men, 20–39 years	0.20–1.10	47.46	0.12
Creatinine (mg/dl)			
Men and women, 50–80 years	0.52–1.08	18.95	0.15
Men, 20–39 years	0.65–1.11	14.31	0.13
Uric acid (mg/dl)			
Men and women, 50–80 years	3.19–7.30	21.51	1.32
Men, 20–39 years	3.40–7.20	19.05	1.23
Total cholesterol (mg/dl)			
Men and women, 50–80 years	173.1–298.1	14.43	32.7
Men, 20–39 years	124.0–256.0	18.10	19.7
Glucose fasting (mg/dl)			
Men and women, 50–80 years	79–129	12.47	16.3
Men, 20–39 years	71–114	11.42	11.0

feasible, meaningful, and desirable that an experienced clinician in everyday practice should have an integrative view of medical findings, in clinical pharmacological studies there is an increasing tendency toward a rigid assessment of study results — which in turn calls for an alignment of reference ranges. This has occurred partially under the influence of quality-assurance officers operating in (perhaps too) strict accordance with the guidelines of good clinical practice, but also as a correct consequence of uncritical interpretations of clinical results by inexperienced investigators.

However, even when using age-related reference ranges, two important aspects must always be remembered: (a) The concept of reference ranges is a statistical one which encompasses the central 95% of all values in the reference sample group. Thus 5% of all values of a healthy population must by definition fall outside the reference limits, and if many tests are performed — as often in prestudy screening — the number of test results outside the reference limits must increase. (b) Biological and chronological age are not the same: only chronological age can be assessed exactly, but not the biological age, which, however, is the relevant factor that influences reference ranges.

Table 114. Reference ranges and coefficient of variation of hematological variables, young and elderly subjects

	Reference range	CV (%)
Leukocytes (10^9/l)		
Men and women, 50–80 years	4.8–10.4	22.40
Men, 20–39 years	4.3–10.7	25.22
Erythrocytes (10^6/μl)		
Men and women, 50–80 years	3.94–5.32	8.05
Men, 20–39 years	4.28–5.60	7.36
Hemoglobin (g/dl)		
Men and women, 50–80 years	11.4–16.3	9.32
Men, 20–39 years	12.8–16.9	6.98
Hematocrit (%)		
Men and women, 50–80 years	34.4–49.0	8.64
Men, 20–39 years	37.6–50.4	7.58
Platelets (10^9/l)		
Men and women, 50–80 years	156–405	24.24
Men, 20–39 years	170–343	18.81
Lymphocytes (%)		
Men and women, 50–80 years	20–49	23.27
Men, 20–39 years	25–55	20.75
Segmented neutrophils (%)		
Men and women, 50–80 years	44–75	13.65
Men, 20–39 years	39–72	15.18
Quick's test (%)		
Men and women, 50–80 years	93–138	10.35
Men, 20–39 years	82–130	11.46

Important for the interpretation of clinical pharmacological study results are furthermore the changes in parameters during repeated measurements, i.e., in the course of a study day or over subsequent study days, which definitely call for knowledge of normal variation over time. This variation over time is attributable to three components: (a) the preanalytical variation (e.g., tourniquet application, diet, sample handling), (b) the analytical imprecision, i.e., the unavoidable random error of every measurement, and (c) the inherent biological variation, which can be regarded as random fluctuation around an individual homeostatic setting point. This intrasubject variability is expressed in the present data as reference range of changes (i.e., the central 95% range of all observed changes) and as Dcrit. The two methods adopt different approaches and are based on different assumptions, but in the main they produce similar results. In the case of repeated measurements or control examinations, both methods denote the changes in a parameter, above which it can be assumed that the observed changes exceed biological and methodological variations.

Our data clearly demonstrate the following: (a) The means are surprisingly stable, even over relatively long observation periods. (b) Individual intrasubject variability over time is, however, greater than most clinical pharmacologists and clinicians would assume (Tables 111, 113). (c) Intrasubject variability over time is in most cases not similar in young and elderly subjects, as postulated from studies in elderly patients, but is often more pronounced in elderly subjects than in the young. This is true for both blood pressure (Table 111) and for many clinical chemistry (Table 113) and hematological variables (Table 114). One notable, but not surprising, finding is that the intrasubject variability of ambulatory 24-h blood pressure monitoring is approximately only half as large as is the case with conventional blood pressure office measurements, even under standardized conditions.

Variations over time are furthermore dependent on baseline values of the parameters in question, i.e., they are often smallest with medium baseline values but greater with baseline values near the limits of the reference ranges (Tables 115, 116). Moreover, these variations depend on sex, (Table 117) and on the length of the period between two repeated measurements, which should be kept in mind when planning clinical trials and analyzing the study results.

Table 115. D_{crit} as function of baseline value (lowest, middle, highest thirds) of blood pressure and pulse rate, men and women aged 50–80 years

	D_{crit}
Systolic BP	
All	13.61
Lowest third	12.04
Middle third	13.56
Highest third	12.01
Diastolic BP	
All	11.52
Lowest third	9.85
Middle third	7.25
Highest third	10.83
Pulse rate	
All	18.07
Lowest third	15.36
Middle third	10.85
Highest third	18.65

Table 116. D_{crit} as function of baseline value (lowest, middle, highest thirds) of clinical chemistry parameters (conventional units)

	Elderly subjects	Young subjects
Alkaline phosphatase		
All	15.30	13.16
Lowest third	11.60	11.09
Middle third	12.97	13.58
Highest third	18.40	15.28
AST (SGOT)		
All	4.70	3.04
Lowest third	2.04	2.19
Middle third	2.94	2.98
Highest third	4.46	3.29
ALT (SGPT)		
All	3.63	3.57
Lowest third	1.88	1.75
Middle third	3.26	3.17
Highest third	5.14	3.92

Table 116. (continued)

	Elderly subjects	Young subjects
γ-GT		
All	4.14	2.37
Lowest third	0.61	1.43
Middle third	3.36	1.99
Highest third	3.69	2.40
LDH		
All	48.70	33.24
Lowest third	34.66	25.28
Middle third	34.06	18.69
Highest third	50.44	38.22
Total bilirubin		
All	0.27	0.12
Lowest third	0.19	0.11
Middle third	0.26	0.12
Highest third	0.30	0.12
Creatinine		
All	0.15	0.13
Lowest third	0.11	0.12
Middle third	0.17	0.12
Highest third	0.14	0.13
Uric acid		
All	1.32	1.23
Lowest third	0.87	0.99
Middle third	1.08	1.04
Highest third	1.48	1.14
Total cholesterol		
All	32.70	19.73
Lowest third	18.39	11.60
Middle third	26.41	18.42
Highest third	34.80	22.47
Triglycerides		
All	20.30	nd
Lowest third	18.42	nd
Middle third	22.71	nd
Highest third	20.42	nd
Glucose fasting		
All	16.30	10.95
Lowest third	11.72	9.57
Middle third	14.10	8.35
Highest third	14.38	9.61

nd, Not determined

Table 117. Differences of D_{crit} in clinical chemistry parameters after 1 week between men and women (conventional units)

	Men and women, 50–80 years	Men, 50–80 years	Women, 50–80 years
Alkaline phosphatase	15.3	15.2	15.0
AST (SGOT)	4.7	4.5	4.8
ALT (SGPT)	3.6	3.2	3.8
γ-GT	4.1	4.3	4.2
LDH	48.7	49.3	48.4
Total bilirubin	0.27	0.31	0.25
Creatinine	0.15	0.17	0.14
Uric acid	1.32	1.40	1.14
Total cholesterol	32.7	30.4	34.3
Triglycerides	20.3	11.7	32.8
Glucose fasting	16.3	12.1	20.2

6 Statistical Details

6.1 Blood Pressure

6.1.1 Baseline Values

6.1.1.1 Elderly Subjects

Table 118. Blood pressure and pulse rate: baseline, **men and women** aged 50–80 years (8:00–9:00 A.M.)

	n	Mean	SD	CI-Up.	CI-Lo.	Med.	Max.	Min.	Lo.Qt.	Up.Qt.	RR-Lo.L	RR-Up.L
Supine												
Systolic BP (mmHg)	1187	129.39	17.40	130.38	128.40	128	186	88	118	140	100	168
Diastolic BP (mmHg)	1187	78.93	9.54	79.47	78.38	80	108	50	72	85	60	98
Pulse rate (bpm)	1187	68.86	9.12	69.38	68.34	68	108	44	62	74	52	88
Standing												
Systolic BP (mmHg)	1050	127.80	17.57	128.87	126.74	126	188	82	116	140	98	168
Diastolic BP (mmHg)	1050	81.54	10.05	82.15	80.93	80	114	58	76	88	60	102
Pulse rate (bpm)	1050	76.42	10.22	77.04	75.80	76	122	43	69	84	60	98
Diff. (standing-supine)												
Systolic BP (mmHg)	1050	−2.53	10.83	−1.88	−3.19	−2	42	−46	−8	4	−26	20
Diastolic BP (mmHg)	1050	2.32	7.17	2.75	1.89	2	28	−20	−2	8	−12	20
Pulse rate (bpm)	1050	8.05	7.49	8.50	7.60	8	38	−44	4	12	−7	25
Age (years)	1187	67.6	6.2	–	–	–	80	50	–	–	–	–

SD, Standard deviation; *CI-Up.*, 95% upper confidence limit; *CI-Lo.*, 95% lower confidence limit; *Med.*, median; *Max.*, maximum; *Min.*, minimum; *Lo.Q.*, lower quartile; *Up.Qt.*, upper quartile; *RR-Lo.L*, lower limit of reference range; *RR-Up.L*, upper limit of reference range.

Table 119. Blood pressure and pulse rate: baseline, **men** aged 50–80 years

	n	Mean	SD	CI-Up.	CI-Lo.	Med.	Max.	Min.	Lo.Qt.	Up.Qt.	RR-Lo.L	RR-Up.L
Supine												
Systolic BP (mmHg)	551	129.15	16.66	130.54	127.75	128	184	88	118	140	100	162
Diastolic BP (mmHg)	551	79.62	9.28	80.39	78.84	80	104	58	72	86	64	98
Pulse rate (bpm)	551	67.79	8.80	68.53	67.06	68	100	47	61	73	52	87
Standing												
Systolic BP (mmHg)	536	127.54	17.44	129.02	126.06	126	188	82	116	140	98	168
Diastolic BP (mmHg)	536	82.06	9.82	82.89	81.23	81	114	60	76	90	62	102
Pulse rate (bpm)	536	76.35	10.17	77.21	75.49	76	116	44	69	84	59	98
Diff. (standing-supine)												
Systolic BP (mmHg)	536	-1.57	10.47	-0.69	-2.46	-2	42	-32	-6	4	-24	22
Diastolic BP (mmHg)	536	2.37	7.19	2.98	1.76	2	28	-20	-2	8	-12	18
Pulse rate (bpm)	536	8.48	6.86	9.06	7.90	8	38	-22	4	12	-6	23
Age (years)	551	67.5	6.1	–	–	–	80	50	–	–	–	–

SD, Standard deviation; *CI-Up.*, 95% upper confidence limit; *CI-Lo.*, 95% lower confidence limit; *Med.*, median; *Max.*, maximum; *Min.*, minimum; *Lo.Q.*, lower quartile; *Up.Qt.*, upper quartile; *RR-Lo.*, lower limit of reference range; *RR-Up.*, upper limit of reference range.

Table 120. Blood pressure and pulse rate: baseline, **women** aged 50–80 years (8:00–9:00 A.M.)

	n	Mean	SD	CI-Up.	CI-Lo.	Med.	Max.	Min.	Lo.Qt.	Up.Qt.	RR-Lo.L	RR-Up.L
Supine												
Systolic BP (mmHg)	636	129.60	18.02	131.00	128.20	128	186	88	116	142	100	168
Diastolic BP (mmHg)	636	78.33	9.72	79.08	77.57	78	108	50	72	84	60	98
Pulse rate (bpm)	636	69.78	9.29	70.51	69.06	68	108	44	64	76	54	91
Standing												
Systolic BP (mmHg)	514	128.08	17.72	129.61	126.55	126	188	88	118	140	98	168
Diastolic BP (mmHg)	514	81.00	10.27	81.89	80.11	80	110	58	74	88	60	102
Pulse rate (bpm)	514	76.49	10.29	77.38	75.60	76	122	43	69	83	60	98
Diff. (standing-supine)												
Systolic BP (mmHg)	514	-3.54	11.11	-2.57	-4.50	-4	42	-46	-10	4	-28	20
Diastolic BP (mmHg)	514	2.26	7.16	2.88	1.64	2	28	-20	-2	6	-12	18
Pulse rate (bpm)	514	7.60	8.07	8.30	6.90	7	33	-44	3	12	-7	25
Age (years)	636	67.7	6.2	–	–	–	80	50	–	–	–	–

SD, Standard deviation; *CI-Up.*, 95% upper confidence limit; *CI-Lo.*, 95% lower confidence limit; *Med.*, median; *Max.*, maximum; *Min.*, minimum; *Lo.Q.*, lower quartile; *Up.Qt.*, upper quartile; *RR-Lo.L*, lower limit of reference range; *RR-Up.L*, upper limit of reference range.

Table 121. Blood pressure and pulse rate: baseline, **men and women** aged 50–59 years (8:00–9:00 A.M.)

	n	Mean	SD	CI-Up.	CI-Lo.	Med.	Max.	Min.	Lo.Qt.	Up.Qt.	RR-Lo.L	RR-Up.L
Supine												
Systolic BP (mmHg)	311	121.78	15.87	123.55	120.02	118	184	88	112	130	98	160
Diastolic BP (mmHg)	311	77.51	9.54	78.57	76.45	78	104	50	70	84	60	98
Pulse rate (bpm)	311	68.29	8.56	69.24	67.34	68	100	50	62	73	55	88
Standing												
Systolic BP (mmHg)	243	121.14	16.90	123.26	119.02	120	188	88	110	130	96	168
Diastolic BP (mmHg)	243	80.37	10.59	81.70	79.04	80	114	58	74	88	60	100
Pulse rate (bpm)	243	74.97	9.79	76.20	73.74	74	116	54	68	80	60	96
Diff. (standing-supine)												
Systolic BP (mmHg)	243	-2.32	9.47	-1.13	-3.51	-2	42	-46	-6	2	-20	18
Diastolic BP (mmHg)	243	2.13	6.52	2.95	1.31	2	22	-20	-2	8	-12	14
Pulse rate (bpm)	243	8.07	7.28	8.99	7.16	8	28	-22	3	12	-8	17
Age (years)	311	57.3	2.2	–	–	–	59	50	–	–	–	–

SD, Standard deviation; CI-Up, 95% upper confidence limit; CI-Lo, 95% lower confidence limit; Med, median; Max, maximum; Min, minimum; Lo.Q, lower quartile; Up.Qt, upper quartile; RR-Lo.L, lower limit of reference range; RR-Up.L, upper limit of reference range.

Table 122. Blood pressure and pulse rate: baseline, **men and women** aged 60–69 years (8:00–9:00 A.M.)

	n	Mean	SD	CI-Up.	CI-Lo.	Med.	Max.	Min.	Lo.Qt.	Up.Qt.	RR-Lo.L	RR-Up.L
Supine												
Systolic BP (mmHg)	652	129.79	16.36	131.04	128.53	129	178	88	120	140	100	164
Diastolic BP (mmHg)	652	79.35	9.24	80.06	78.64	80	104	52	72	86	60	98
Pulse rate (bpm)	652	68.40	9.18	69.11	67.70	68	108	44	62	74	52	88
Standing												
Systolic BP (mmHg)	587	127.27	16.78	128.63	125.92	126	180	82	118	138	100	150
Diastolic BP (mmHg)	587	81.95	10.02	82.76	81.13	80	112	58	76	90	62	96
Pulse rate (bpm)	587	75.93	10.05	76.75	75.12	76	122	48	68	83	59	95
Diff. (standing-supine)												
Systolic BP (mmHg)	587	-2.57	10.86	-1.69	-3.44	-2	42	-38	-8	4	-26	10
Diastolic BP (mmHg)	587	2.52	7.11	3.10	1.95	2	28	-20	4	0	-12	12
Pulse rate (bpm)	587	7.93	7.23	8.51	7.34	8	33	-22	4	12	-7	17
Age (years)	652	67.0	2.9	–	–	–	69	60	–	–	–	–

SD, Standard deviation; *CI-Up.*, 95% upper confidence limit; *CI-Lo.*, 95% lower confidence limit; *Med.*, median; *Max*, maximum; *Min.*, minimum; *Lo.Q.*, lower quartile; *Up.Qt.*, upper quartile; *RR-Lo.L*, lower limit of reference range; *RR-Up.L*, upper limit of reference range.

Table 123. Blood pressure and pulse rate: baseline, **men and women** aged 70–80 years (8:00–9:00 A.M.)

	n	Mean	SD	CI-Up.	CI-Lo.	Med.	Max.	Min.	Lo.Qt.	Up.Qt.	RR-Lo.L	RR-Up.L
Supine												
Systolic BP (mmHg)	224	138.78	17.57	141.08	136.48	138	186	90	128	152	106	172
Diastolic BP (mmHg)	224	79.66	10.22	80.99	78.32	80	108	58	72	86	62	100
Pulse rate (bpm)	224	70.98	9.42	72.21	69.74	71	100	47	64	78	52	89
Standing												
Systolic BP (mmHg)	220	136.58	16.81	138.80	134.36	138	188	90	124	148	104	174
Diastolic BP (mmHg)	220	81.76	9.45	83.01	80.51	80	110	58	76	90	64	102
Pulse rate (bpm)	220	79.31	10.63	80.72	77.91	80	102	43	72	87	58	100
Diff. (standing-supine)												
Systolic BP (mmHg)	220	−2.68	12.10	−1.08	−4.28	−3	26	−40	−10	6	−28	20
Diastolic BP (mmHg)	220	1.98	8.00	3.04	0.92	2	28	−20	−4	8	−16	18
Pulse rate (bpm)	220	8.35	8.36	9.46	7.25	7	38	−44	4	12	−5	30
Age (years)	224	74.9	2.9	–	–	–	80	70	–	–	–	–

SD, Standard deviation; *CI-Up.*, 95% upper confidence limit; *CI-Lo.*, 95% lower confidence limit; *Med.*, median; *Max.*, maximum; *Min.*, minimum; *Lo.Q.*, lower quartile; *Up.Qt.*, upper quartile; *RR-Lo.L*, lower limit of reference range; *RR-Up.L*, upper limit of reference range.

6.1.1.2 Young Subjects

Table 124. Blood pressure and pulse rate: baseline, **men** aged 20–39 years (8:00–9:00 A.M.)

	n	Mean	SD	CI-Up.	CI-Lo.	Med.	Max.	Min.	Lo.Qt.	Up.Qt.	RR-Lo.L	RR-Up.L
Supine												
Systolic BP (mmHg)	1265	119.10	10.47	119.67	118.52	120	170	90	112	124	100	142
Diastolic BP (mmHg)	1265	73.77	7.65	74.19	73.35	72	100	48	70	80	60	90
Pulse rate (bpm)	1265	65.21	8.76	65.69	64.73	64	102	38	60	71	50	84
Standing												
Systolic BP (mmHg)	757	117.30	10.70	118.07	116.54	116	156	84	110	124	100	142
Diastolic BP (mmHg)	757	77.34	8.33	77.94	76.75	78	102	58	70	82	62	98
Pulse rate (bpm)	757	77.75	10.39	78.49	77.00	76	108	44	71	85	60	100
Diff. (standing-supine)												
Systolic BP (mmHg)	757	-2.82	7.61	-2.28	-3.36	-2	24	-34	-8	2	-18	12
Diastolic BP (mmHg)	757	3.94	7.13	4.45	3.43	4	38	-20	0	8	-10	18
Pulse rate (bpm)	757	12.58	8.98	13.22	11.94	10	44	-28	7	18	-2	33
Age (years)	1265	27.2	4.2	-	-	-	39	20	-	-	-	-

SD, Standard deviation; *CI-Up.*, 95% upper confidence limit; *CI-Lo.*, 95% lower confidence limit; *Med.*, median; *Max.*, maximum; *Min.*, minimum; *Lo.Q.*, lower quartile; *Up.Qt.*, upper quartile; *RR-Lo.L*, lower limit of reference range; *RR-Up.L*, upper limit of reference range.

Table 125. Blood pressure and pulse rate: baseline, **men** aged 20–29 years (8:00–9:00 A.M.)

	n	Mean	SD	CI-Up.	CI-Lo.	Med.	Max.	Min.	Lo.Qt.	Up.Qt.	RR-Lo.L	RR-Up.L
Supine												
Systolic BP (mmHg)	900	119.37	10.54	120.06	118.69	120	170	90	112	126	100	142
Diastolic BP (mmHg)	900	73.51	7.55	74.00	73.01	72	98	48	68	80	60	90
Pulse rate (bpm)	900	65.21	8.81	65.78	64.63	64	102	38	60	71	50	85
Standing												
Systolic BP (mmHg)	550	117.38	10.10	118.22	116.54	118	156	90	110	124	100	138
Diastolic BP (mmHg)	550	77.29	8.07	77.97	76.62	78	102	58	70	82	62	92
Pulse rate (bpm)	550	78.20	10.55	79.08	77.32	78	108	44	72	85	60	98
Diff. (standing-supine)												
Systolic BP (mmHg)	550	−2.89	7.49	−2.27	−3.52	−4	24	−30	−8	2	−18	10
Diastolic BP (mmHg)	550	4.08	7.01	4.67	3.50	4	28	−20	0	8	−8	18
Pulse rate (bpm)	550	12.93	9.31	13.71	12.15	12	44	−28	7	18	−2	31
Age (years)	900	25.0	2.2	–	–	–	29	20	–	–	–	–

SD, Standard deviation; *CI-Up.*, 95% upper confidence limit; *CI-Lo.*, 95% lower confidence limit; *Med.*, median; *Max.*, maximum; *Min.*, minimum; *Lo.Q.*, lower quartile; *Up.Qt.*, upper quartile; *RR-Lo.L*, lower limit of reference range; *RR-Up.L*, upper limit of reference range.

Table 126. Blood pressure and pulse rate: baseline, **men** aged 30–39 years (8:00–9:00 A.M.)

	n	Mean	SD	CI-Up.	CI-Lo.	Med.	Max.	Min.	Lo.Qt.	Up.Qt.	RR-Lo.L	RR-Up.L
Supine												
Systolic BP (mmHg)	365	118.41	10.29	119.47	117.36	118	150	94	110	124	100	140
Diastolic BP (mmHg)	365	74.43	7.86	75.23	73.62	74	100	58	70	80	60	90
Pulse rate (bpm)	365	65.21	8.64	66.10	64.33	64	96	44	60	70	48	83
Standing												
Systolic BP (mmHg)	207	117.10	12.18	118.76	115.44	116	152	84	110	124	98	144
Diastolic BP (mmHg)	207	77.49	8.99	78.71	76.26	78	100	60	70	84	60	98
Pulse rate (bpm)	207	76.54	9.87	77.88	75.19	75	102	56	69	84	60	96
Diff. (standing-supine)												
Systolic BP (mmHg)	207	-2.62	7.93	-1.54	-3.70	-2	22	-34	-8	2	-18	14
Diastolic BP (mmHg)	207	3.57	7.43	4.58	2.55	4	38	-18	-2	8	-10	22
Pulse rate (bpm)	207	11.65	7.98	12.73	10.56	9	34	-4	6	16	0	33
Age (years)	365	32.76	2.46	–	–	–	39	30	–	–	–	–

SD, Standard deviation; *CI-Up.*, 95% upper confidence limit; *CI-Lo.*, 95% lower confidence limit; *Med.*, median; *Max.*, maximum; *Min.*, minimum; *Lo.Q.*, lower quartile; *Up.Qt.*, upper quartile; *RR-Lo.L*, lower limit of reference range; *RR-Up.L*, upper limit of reference range.

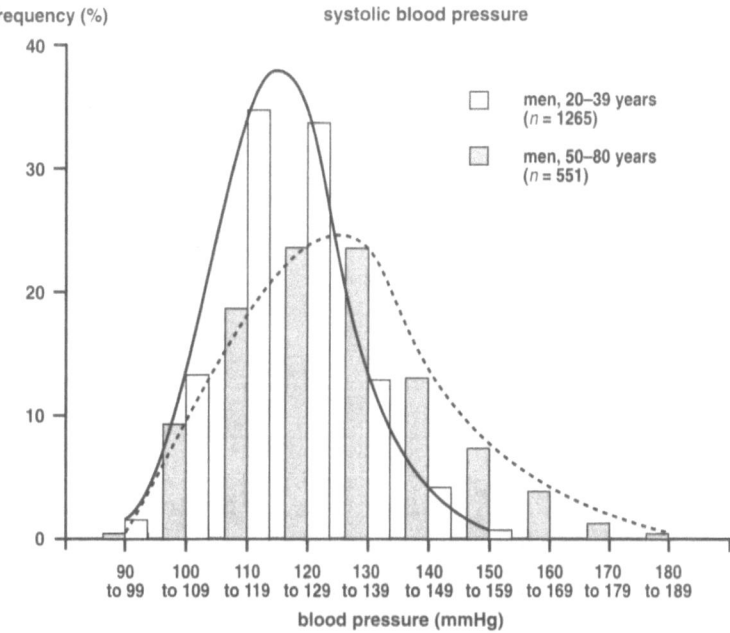

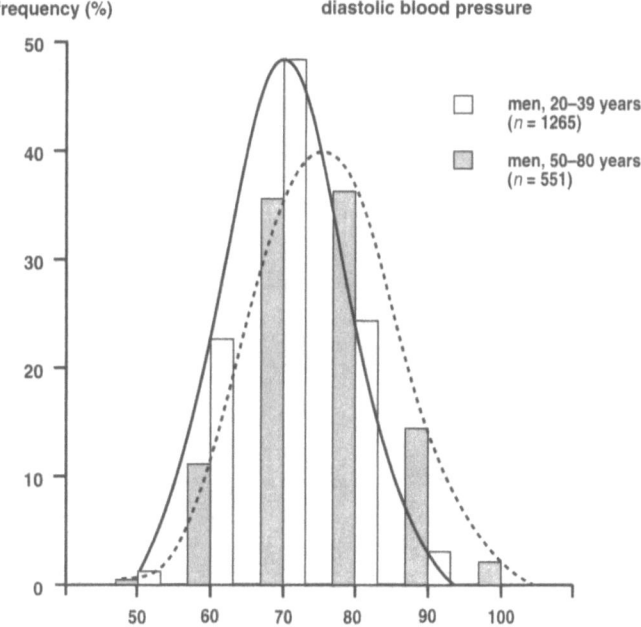

Fig. 6. Frequency distribution of supine systolic and diastolic blood pressure in young men (20–39 years) and men aged 50–80 years

6.1.2 Changes During Study Day

6.1.2.1 Elderly Subjects

Table 127. Blood pressure and pulse rate, supine: changes during study day, differences from baseline, **men and women** aged 50–80 years

	n	Mean	SD	CI-Up.	CI-Lo.	Med.	Min.	Max.	Lo.Qt.	Up.Qt.	RR-Lo.L	RR-Up.L	D$_{crit}$
2 h													
Systolic BP (mmHg)	141	0.21	12.30	2.24	-1.82	0	-34	32	-8	8	-22	24	25.7
Diastolic BP (mmHg)	141	-1.45	8.35	-0.08	-2.83	-2	-26	26	-8	4	-16	14	16.1
Pulse rate (bpm)	141	-2.31	8.49	-0.91	-3.71	-2	-28	18	-8	4	-20	12	16.4
4 h													
Systolic BP (mmHg)	210	-0.94	12.29	0.72	-2.61	0	-26	24	-10	8	-24	20	23.8
Diastolic BP (mmHg)	210	-1.11	9.21	0.14	-2.35	0	-22	28	-8	4	-20	18	18.0
Pulse rate (bpm)	210	-1.06	9.37	0.21	-2.33	-1	-22	48	-6	4	-18	16	18.4
6 h													
Systolic BP (mmHg)	168	-2.18	11.92	-0.38	-3.99	-4	-28	28	-12	6	-22	22	23.0
Diastolic BP (mmHg)	168	-4.16	9.45	-2.73	-5.59	-4	-34	22	-10	2	-24	14	18.8
Pulse rate (bpm)	168	3.26	10.78	4.89	1.63	4	-35	34	-3	10	-21	23	21.4
10 h													
Systolic BP (mmHg)	128	-1.16	12.54	1.01	-3.34	0	-34	24	-10	8	-26	22	23.5
Diastolic BP (mmHg)	128	-2.21	10.56	-0.38	-4.04	-2	-28	30	-10	4	-24	18	20.3
Pulse rate (bpm)	128	2.48	10.01	4.22	0.75	3	-18	22	-6	12	-16	18	22.7
Age (years)	210	66.6	5.4	–	–	–	53	77	–	–	–	–	–

SD, Standard deviation; *CI-Up.*, 95% upper confidence limit; *CI-Lo.*, 95% lower confidence limit; *Med.*, median; *Max.*, maximum; *Min.*, minimum; *Lo.Q.*, lower quartile; *Up.Qt.*, upper quartile; *RR-Lo.L*, lower limit of reference range; *RR-Up.L*, upper limit of reference range; *D$_{crit}$*, critical difference 0.05.

6.1.2.2 Young Subjects

Table 128. Blood pressure and pulse rate, supine: changes during study day, differences from baseline, **men** aged 20–39

	n	Mean	SD	CI-Up.	CI-Lo.	Med.	Min.	Max.	Lo.Qt.	Up.Qt.	RR-Lo.L	RR-Up.L	D_{crit}
2 h													
Systolic BP (mmHg)	287	-1.16	5.58	-0.52	-1.81	-2	-16	12	-6	2	-10	10	12.8
Diastolic BP (mmHg)	287	0.40	6.03	1.09	-0.30	0	-16	18	-4	4	-12	12	10.7
Pulse rate (bpm)	287	-2.92	7.19	-2.08	-3.75	-2	-23	20	-8	2	-19	10	11.5
4 h													
Systolic BP (mmHg)	233	0.94	6.76	1.81	0.08	2	-18	16	-4	6	-12	14	14.5
Diastolic BP (mmHg)	233	-0.22	6.03	0.56	-0.99	0	-14	14	-4	4	-10	12	11.9
Pulse rate (bpm)	233	1.69	8.45	2.77	0.60	2	-22	23	-4	8	-14	19	16.8
6 h													
Systolic BP (mmHg)	254	0.24	7.31	1.14	-0.66	0	-16	18	-6	6	-12	16	10.6
Diastolic BP (mmHg)	254	-1.55	6.39	-0.76	-2.33	-2	-16	12	-6	4	-12	12	13.0
Pulse rate (bpm)	254	0.98	7.32	1.88	0.08	1	-14	20	-4	6	-12	15	14.0
10 h													
Systolic BP (mmHg)	226	2.08	7.69	3.09	1.08	2	-20	18	-2	8	-12	16	17.0
Diastolic BP (mmHg)	226	-1.16	6.13	-0.36	-1.96	-2	-14	18	-6	2	-12	12	13.1
Pulse rate (bpm)	226	2.19	7.43	3.16	1.22	3	-17	20	-2	7	-12	16	15.0
Age (years)	287	27.0	4.2	–	–	–	20	39	–	–	–	–	–

SD, Standard deviation; *CI-Up.*, 95% upper confidence limit; *CI-Lo*, 95% lower confidence limit; *Med.*, median; *Max.*, maximum; *Min.*, minimum; *Lo.Q*, lower quartile; *Up.Qt.*, upper quartile; *RR-Lo.L*, lower limit of reference range; *RR-Up.L*, upper limit of reference range; *D_crit*, critical difference 0.05.

6.1.3 Changes After Repeated Measurements

6.1.3.1 Elderly Subjects

Table 129. Blood pressure and pulse rate: changes **after 24 h**, differences from baseline, men and women aged 50–80

	n	Mean	SD	CI-Up.	CI-Lo.	Med.	Max.	Min.	RR-Lo.L	RR-Up.L	D_{crit}
Supine											
Systolic BP (mmHg)	180	0.42	3.38	0.91	-0.08	0	8	-10	-6	6	6.6
Diastolic BP (mmHg)	180	-0.46	3.96	0.12	-1.03	0	10	-10	-8	8	7.1
Pulse rate (bpm)	180	-0.03	4.58	0.64	-0.70	0	15	-14	-8	11	8.5
Standing											
Systolic BP (mmHg)	180	-0.22	5.35	0.56	-1.00	0	16	-14	-10	12	10.8
Diastolic BP (mmHg)	180	0.03	6.39	0.97	-0.90	0	24	-16	-12	14	12.4
Pulse rate (bpm)	180	0.16	6.67	1.13	-0.81	0	18	-14	-12	16	12.2
Age (years)	180	66.1	5.0	–	–	–	80	56	–	–	–

SD, Standard deviation; *CI-Up.*, 95% upper confidence limit; *CI-Lo.*, 95% lower confidence limit; *Med.*, median; *Max.*, maximum; *Min.*, minimum; *RR-Lo.L*, lower limit of reference range; *RR-Up.L*, upper limit of reference range; D_{crit} critical difference 0.05.

Table 130. Blood pressure and pulse rate: changes **after 48 h**, differences from baseline, men and women aged 50–80 years

	n	Mean	SD	CI-Up.	CI-Lo.	Med.	Max.	Min.	RR-Lo.L	RR-Up.L	D_{crit}
Supine											
Systolic BP (mmHg)	123	1.85	9.90	3.60	0.10	0	24	-16	-14	20	18.0
Diastolic BP (mmHg)	123	-1.06	8.57	0.46	-2.57	-2	22	-22	-16	16	15.8
Pulse rate (bpm)	123	-0.01	8.13	1.43	-1.44	0	18	-24	-17	16	16.2
Standing											
Systolic BP (mmHg)	123	-0.53	11.83	1.56	-2.62	-2	34	-24	-20	24	22.1
Diastolic BP (mmHg)	123	-1.69	8.47	-0.19	-3.19	-2	22	-20	-16	16	17.2
Pulse rate (bpm)	123	-1.20	8.57	0.32	-2.71	0	14	-26	-18	14	15.9
Age (years)	123	65.9	6.1	–	–	–	80	51	–	–	–

SD, Standard deviation; *CI-Up.*, 95% upper confidence limit; *CI-Lo.*, 95% lower confidence limit; *Med.*, median; *Max.*, maximum; *Min.*, minimum; *RR-Lo.L*, lower limit of reference range; *RR-Up.L*, upper limit of reference range; D_{crit} critical difference 0.05.

Table 131. Blood pressure and pulse rate: changes **after 1 week**, differences from baseline, men and women aged 50–80 years

	n	Mean	SD	CI-Up.	CI-Lo.	Med.	Max.	Min.	RR-Lo.L	RR-Up.L	D_{crit}
Supine											
Systolic BP (mmHg)	229	-0.83	7.15	0.09	-1.76	-2	20	-16	-12	13	13.6
Diastolic BP (mmHg)	229	-1.34	5.88	-0.57	-2.10	-2	12	-16	-12	10	11.5
Pulse rate (bpm)	229	-1.38	9.67	-0.13	-2.63	-1	37	-36	-16	16	18.1
Standing											
Systolic BP (mmHg)	219	-1.61	11.19	-0.13	-3.09	-2	32	-32	-18	16	21.8
Diastolic BP (mmHg)	219	-0.20	7.70	0.82	-1.22	0	18	-20	-14	14	15.9
Pulse rate (bpm)	219	-1.15	10.33	0.22	-2.52	-1	30	-36	-18	26	19.7
Age (years)	229	65.2	6.1	–	–	–	80	51	–	–	–

SD, Standard deviation; *CI-Up.*, 95% upper confidence limit; *CI-Lo.*, 95% lower confidence limit; *Med.*, median; *Max.*, maximum; *Min.*, minimum; *RR-Up.L*, upper limit of reference range; *RR-Lo.L*, lower limit of reference range; D_{crit} critical difference 0.05.

Table 132. Blood pressure and pulse rate: changes **after 2 weeks**, differences from baseline, men and women aged 50–80

n	Mean	SD	CI-Up.	CI-Lo.	Med.	Max.	Min.	RR-Lo.L	RR-Up.L	D_{crit}
Supine										
Systolic BP (mmHg)	211	-1.00	8.59	0.16	-2.15	-2	20	-36	-15	14	16.4
Diastolic BP (mmHg)	211	-0.49	8.63	0.68	-1.65	0	20	-23	-14	18	16.9
Pulse rate (bpm)	211	0.14	10.26	1.52	-1.25	1	30	-36	-22	22	20.1
Standing										
Systolic BP (mmHg)	211	-1.65	12.94	0.09	-3.40	0	30	-42	-26	24	25.7
Diastolic BP (mmHg)	211	-0.13	9.84	1.19	-1.46	0	22	-28	-20	18	19.8
Pulse rate (bpm)	211	-0.56	11.14	0.94	-2.06	0	26	-56	-22	22	21.7
Age (years)	211	65.7	6.1	–	–	–	–	80	51	–	–

SD, Standard deviation; *CI-Up.*, 95% upper confidence limit; *CI-Lo.*, 95% lower confidence limit; *Med.*, median; *Max.*, maximum; *Min.*, minimum; *RR-Lo.L*, lower limit of reference range; *RR-Up.L*, upper limit of reference range; D_{crit} critical difference 0.05.

Table 133. Blood pressure and pulse rate: changes **after 3 weeks**, differences from baseline, men and women aged 50–80

n	Mean	SD	CI-Up.	CI-Lo.	Med.	Max.	Min.	RR-Lo.L	RR-Up.L	D_{crit}
Supine										
Systolic BP (mmHg)	246	-0.09	7.94	0.90	-1.09	0	20	-18	-14	16	15.2
Diastolic BP (mmHg)	246	0.30	7.39	1.23	-0.62	0	20	-23	-14	14	14.1
Pulse rate (bpm)	246	0.13	8.52	1.19	-0.94	0	23	-27	-18	18	16.6
Standing										
Systolic BP (mmHg)	227	-2.07	14.67	-0.17	-3.98	-2	34	-40	-29	28	28.8
Diastolic BP (mmHg)	227	0.64	10.55	2.01	-0.73	2	24	-34	-22	18	19.3
Pulse rate (bpm)	227	-0.99	11.00	0.44	-2.42	-1	26	-49	-19	24	21.8
Age (years)	246	66.5	5.9	–	–	–	–	80	53	–	–

SD, Standard deviation; *CI-Up.*, 95% upper confidence limit; *CI-Lo.*, 95% lower confidence limit; *Med.*, median; *Max.*, maximum; *Min.*, minimum; *RR-Lo.L*, lower limit of reference range; *RR-Up.L*, upper limit of reference range; D_{crit} critical difference 0.05.

6.1.3.2 Young Subjects

Table 134. Blood pressure and pulse rate, supine: changes after 24 h and 1 week, differences from baseline, men aged 20–39

	n	Mean	SD	CI-Up.	CI-Lo.	Med.	Max.	Min.	RR-Lo.L	RR-Up.L	D$_{crit}$
24 h											
Systolic BP (mmHg)	144	2.26	5.00	3.07	1.44	4	12	-12	-8	10	10.0
Diastolic BP (mmHg)	144	0.47	4.04	1.13	-0.19	0	10	-12	-8	8	7.7
Pulse rate (bpm)	144	0.31	6.14	1.31	-0.70	2	12	-16	-12	9	12.8
Age (years)	144	27.1	4.0		38	20					
1 week											
Systolic BP (mmHg)	95	0.62	3.32	1.29	-0.05	0	-8	10	-4	8	6.2
Diastolic BP (mmHg)	95	0.16	3.32	0.83	-0.51	0	-10	8	-6	8	6.6
Pulse rate (bpm)	95	-0.19	6.01	1.02	-1.40	0	-12	13	-10	12	10.8
Age (years)	95	26.9	3.9				38	20			

SD, Standard deviation; CI-Up., 95% upper confidence limit; CI-Lo., 95% lower confidence limit; Med., median; Max., maximum; Min., minimum; RR-Lo.L, lower limit of reference range; RR-Up.L, upper limit of reference range; D$_{crit}$, critical difference 0.05.

6.2 Ambulatory Blood Pressure Monitoring

6.2.1 Baseline Values

Table 135. Ambulatory blood pressure monitoring: baseline, normotensive men and women aged 50–80 years (start of registration between 7:00 and 8:00 A.M.)

	n	Mean	SD	CI-Up.	CI-Lo.	Med.	Max.	Min.	Lo.Qt.	Up.Qt.	RR-Lo.L	RR-Up.L
24 h												
Systolic BP	309	125.28	10.84	126.49	124.08	126.0	156.1	96.9	117.1	133.1	107.2	145.3
Diastolic BP	309	75.58	6.65	76.32	74.83	75.2	92.3	59.0	71.1	80.0	63.1	88.2
Day												
Systolic BP	309	129.44	11.23	130.70	128.19	130.0	165.5	101.0	120.1	137.1	110.2	150.3
Diastolic BP	309	79.34	7.10	80.13	78.55	79.9	93.2	59.0	74.1	84.0	66.1	92.2
Night												
Systolic BP	309	119.37	11.72	120.67	118.06	120.1	147.4	92.2	111.0	127.1	97.2	144.3
Diastolic BP	309	70.26	7.19	71.06	69.46	71.2	90.3	54.9	65.2	75.1	57.1	84.2
Age (years)	309	66.9	4.5	–	–	–	80	57	–	–	–	–
Office measurements												
Systolic BP Supine	232	128.69	16.92	130.87	126.51	129	201	86	–	–	–	–
Diastolic BP Supine	232	77.32	10.52	78.68	75.97	77	99	47	–	–	–	–

Office measurements, immediately before start of ABPM; *SD*, standard deviation; *CI-Up.*, 95% upper confidence limit; *CI-Lo.*, 95% lower confidence limit; *Med.*, median; *Max.*, maximum; *Min.*, minimum; *Lo.Q.*, lower quartile; *Up.Qt.*, upper quartile; *RR-Lo.L*, lower limit of reference range; *RR-Up.L*, upper limit of reference range.

Table 136. Ambulatory blood pressure monitoring; baseline, hypertensive men and women aged 50–80 years (start of registration between 7:00 and 8:00 A.M.)

	n	Mean	SD	CI-Up.	CI-Lo.	Med.	Max.	Min.	RR-Lo.L	RR-Up.L
24 h										
Systolic BP	157	152.72	12.80	154.73	150.72	151.1	198.3	123.8	129.7	179.9
Diastolic BP	157	97.25	7.57	98.43	96.07	96.6	129.8	80.2	85.4	109.5
Day										
Systolic BP	157	159.06	12.89	161.07	157.04	157.1	203.0	130.1	136.9	187.5
Diastolic BP	157	107.97	6.10	108.92	107.02	107.5	123.5	95.0	98.5	119.0
Night										
Systolic BP	157	144.93	14.20	147.15	142.71	144.6	192.8	112.8	119.7	174.2
Diastolic BP	157	89.90	8.65	91.25	88.55	89.8	127.2	71.6	76.2	102.6
Age (years)	157	64.6	4.4	–	–	–	76	60	–	–
Office measurements										
Systolic BP Supine	157	165.66	15.58	168.10	163.22	166	203	131	140	197
Diastolic BP Supine	157	109.75	11.84	111.60	107.90	108	136	95	96	124

Office measurements, immediately before start of ABPM; *SD*, standard deviation; *CI-Up.*, 95% upper confidence limit; *CI-Lo.*, 95% lower confidence limit; *Med.*, median; *Max.*, maximum; *Min.*, minimum; *RR-Lo.L*, lower limit of reference range; *RR-Up.L*, upper limit of reference range.

6.2.2 Changes After 2 Weeks

Table 137. Ambulatory blood pressure monitoring: changes after 2 weeks, differences from baseline, healthy men and women aged 50–80 years (start of registration between 7:00 and 8:00 A.M.)

	n	Mean	SD	CI-Up.	CI-Lo.	Med.	Max.	Min.	RR-Lo.L	RR-Up.L	D_{crit}
24 h											
Systolic BP	101	-0.62	4.79	0.31	-1.55	-1.0	15.0	-8.0	-8.1	8.0	9.6
Diastolic BP	101	-1.04	4.18	-0.22	-1.86	-1.0	9.1	-13.1	-8.0	7.2	8.4
Day											
Systolic BP	101	-0.92	4.61	-0.02	-1.82	-1.0	9.2	-9.1	-8.0	8.1	9.3
Diastolic BP	101	-0.72	4.10	0.08	-1.52	-1.0	7.9	-9.2	-8.3	8.4	8.4
Night											
Systolic BP	101	0.09	6.15	1.29	-1.11	0.0	21.0	-15.1	-10.2	9.9	12.6
Diastolic BP	101	0.14	5.98	1.31	-1.03	1.0	14.1	-16.1	-9.4	13.2	12.1
Age (years)	101	67.4	5.3	–	–	–	76	55	–	–	–

SD, Standard deviation; *CI-Up.*, 95% upper confidence limit; *CI-Lo.*, 95% lower confidence limit; *Med.*, median; *Max.*, maximum; *Min.*, minimum; *RR-Lo.L*, lower limit of reference range; *RR-Up.L*, upper limit of reference range; D_{crit}, critical difference 0.05.

6.3 ECG Times

6.3.1 Baseline Values

6.3.1.1 Elderly Subjects

Table 138. ECG times: baseline, men and women aged 50–80 years (8:00–9:00 A.M.)

	n	Mean	SD	CI-Up.	CI-Lo.	Med.	Max.	Min.	Lo.Qt.	Up.Qt.	RR-Lo.L	RR-Up.L
RR (s)	655	0.94	0.13	0.95	0.93	0.93	1.44	0.62	0.85	1.02	0.69	1.19
P (s)	486	0.10	0.01	0.11	0.10	0.10	0.18	0.06	0.10	0.11	0.08	0.13
PQ (s)	1198	0.16	0.02	0.16	0.16	0.16	0.22	0.11	0.15	0.18	0.12	0.20
QRS (s)	1197	0.09	0.01	0.09	0.09	0.09	0.13	0.06	0.08	0.10	0.07	0.11
QT (s)	1198	0.39	0.02	0.39	0.39	0.39	0.49	0.32	0.38	0.41	0.35	0.44
QTc (s)	571	0.40	0.02	0.41	0.40	0.40	0.46	0.34	0.39	0.41	0.37	0.44
HR (bpm)	1198	65.80	9.45	66.34	65.27	65	98	41	59	72	50	87
Age (years)	1198	67.2	4.7	–	–	–	80	50	–	–	–	–

SD, Standard deviation; *CI-Up.*, 95% upper confidence limit; *CI-Lo.*, 95% lower confidence limit; *Med.*, median; *Max.*, maximum; *Min.*, minimum; *Lo.Q.*, lower quartile; *Up.Qt.*, upper quartile; *RR-Lo.L*, lower limit of reference range; *RR-Up.L*, upper limit of reference range.

Table 139. ECG times: baseline, men aged 50–80 years (8:00–9:00 A.M.)

	n	Mean	SD	CI-Up.	CI-Lo.	Med.	Max.	Min.	Lo.Qt.	Up.Qt.	RR-Lo.L	RR-Up.L
RR (s)	344	0.96	0.13	0.97	0.95	0.95	1.44	0.66	0.87	1.04	0.73	1.23
P (s)	239	0.11	0.01	0.11	0.10	0.10	0.15	0.08	0.10	0.12	0.08	0.13
PQ (s)	582	0.16	0.02	0.16	0.16	0.16	0.22	0.12	0.15	0.18	0.13	0.21
QRS (s)	581	0.09	0.01	0.09	0.09	0.09	0.13	0.07	0.08	0.10	0.07	0.11
QT (s)	582	0.39	0.02	0.39	0.39	0.39	0.49	0.34	0.38	0.40	0.35	0.44
QTc (s)	298	0.41	0.02	0.41	0.40	0.41	0.46	0.36	0.40	0.42	0.37	0.44
HR (bpm)	582	65.55	8.91	66.28	64.83	64	98	46	59	71	52	87
Age (years)	582	67.6	6.3	–	–	–	80	50	–	–	–	–

SD, Standard deviation; *CI-Up.*, 95% upper confidence limit; *CI-Lo*, 95% lower confidence limit; *Med.*, median; *Max.*, maximum; *Min.*, minimum; *Lo.Q.*, lower quartile; *Up.Qt.*, upper quartile; *RR-Lo.L*, lower limit of reference range; *RR-Up.L*, upper limit of reference range.

Table 140. ECG times: baseline, women aged 50–80 years (8:00–9:00 A.M.)

	n	Mean	SD	CI-Up.	CI-Lo.	Med.	Max.	Min.	Lo.Qt.	Up.Qt.	RR-Lo.L	RR-Up.L
RR (s)	311	0.91	0.13	0.93	0.90	0.91	1.19	0.62	0.83	1.00	0.66	1.16
P (s)	247	0.10	0.02	0.10	0.10	0.10	0.18	0.06	0.10	0.11	0.08	0.13
PQ (s)	616	0.16	0.02	0.17	0.16	0.16	0.22	0.11	0.15	0.18	0.12	0.20
QRS (s)	616	0.09	0.01	0.09	0.09	0.09	0.12	0.06	0.08	0.10	0.07	0.11
QT (s)	616	0.39	0.03	0.39	0.39	0.40	0.47	0.32	0.38	0.41	0.34	0.44
QTc (s)	273	0.40	0.02	0.40	0.40	0.40	0.46	0.34	0.39	0.41	0.36	0.44
HR (bpm)	616	66.04	9.93	66.82	65.25	66	92	41	58	73	49	85
Age (years)	616	67.4	6.2	–	–	–	80	50	–	–	–	–

SD, Standard deviation; *CI-Up.*, 95% upper confidence limit; *CI-Lo*, 95% lower confidence limit; *Med.*, median; *Max.*, maximum; *Min.*, minimum; *Lo.Q.*, lower quartile; *Up.Qt.*, upper quartile; *RR-Lo.L*, lower limit of reference range; *RR-Up.L*, upper limit of reference range.

Table 141. ECG times: baseline, men and women aged 50–59 years (8:00–9:00 A.M.)

	n	Mean	SD	CI-Up.	CI-Lo.	Med.	Max.	Min.	Lo.Qt.	Up.Qt.	RR-Lo.L	RR-Up.L
RR (s)	264	0.91	0.12	0.93	0.90	0.91	1.24	0.66	0.84	0.98	0.69	1.18
P (s)	216	0.10	0.01	0.10	0.10	0.10	0.14	0.06	0.10	0.13	0.08	0.13
PQ (s)	360	0.16	0.02	0.16	0.15	0.15	0.20	0.12	0.14	0.16	0.12	0.20
QRS (s)	360	0.09	0.01	0.09	0.09	0.08	0.10	0.06	0.08	0.09	0.07	0.10
QT (s)	360	0.38	0.02	0.38	0.38	0.38	0.43	0.32	0.37	0.40	0.34	0.43
QTc (s)	360	0.40	0.02	0.40	0.40	0.40	0.46	0.36	0.39	0.41	0.37	0.44
HR (bpm)	360	61.79	7.80	62.59	60.98	61	81	44	56	66	50	80
Age (years)	360	58.1	2.2	–	–	–	59	50	–	–	–	–

SD, Standard deviation; *CI-Up.*, 95% upper confidence limit; *CI-Lo.*, 95% lower confidence limit; *Med.*, median; *Max.*, maximum; *Min.*, minimum; *Lo.Q.*, lower quartile; *Up.Qt.*, upper quartile; *RR-Lo.L*, lower limit of reference range; *RR-Up.L*, upper limit of reference range.

Table 142. ECG times: baseline, men and women aged 60–69 years (8:00–9:00 A.M.)

	n	Mean	SD	CI-Up.	CI-Lo.	Med.	Max.	Min.	Lo.Qt.	Up.Qt.	RR-Lo.L	RR-Up.L
RR (s)	287	0.95	0.13	0.96	0.93	0.95	1.28	0.62	0.86	1.04	0.69	1.16
P (s)	203	0.10	0.01	0.11	0.10	0.10	0.18	0.06	0.10	0.12	0.08	0.13
PQ (s)	623	0.17	0.02	0.17	0.17	0.17	0.22	0.11	0.15	0.18	0.13	0.21
QRS (s)	623	0.09	0.01	0.09	0.09	0.09	0.12	0.06	0.08	0.10	0.07	0.11
QT (s)	623	0.40	0.02	0.40	0.39	0.40	0.48	0.32	0.38	0.41	0.35	0.44
QTc (s)	246	0.41	0.02	0.41	0.40	0.40	0.46	0.35	0.39	0.42	0.37	0.45
HR (bpm)	623	67.39	9.40	68.13	66.65	67	94	44	61	73	51	89
Age (years)	623	68.4	3.0	–	–	–	69	60	–	–	–	–

SD, Standard deviation; *CI-Up.*, 95% upper confidence limit; *CI-Lo.*, 95% lower confidence limit; *Med.*, median; *Max.*, maximum; *Min.*, minimum; *Lo.Q.*, lower quartile; *Up.Qt.*, upper quartile; *RR-Lo.L*, lower limit of reference range; *RR-Up.L*, upper limit of reference range.

Table 143. ECG times: baseline, men and women aged 70–80 years (8:00–9:00 A.M.)

	n	Mean	SD	CI-Up.	CI-Lo.	Med.	Max.	Min.	Lo.Qt.	Up.Qt.	RR-Lo.L	RR-Up.L
RR (s)	104	0.97	0.16	–	–	0.95	1.44	0.62	0.85	1.10	0.68	1.30
P (s)	67	0.10	0.01	–	–	0.10	0.15	0.06	0.10	0.11	0.06	0.13
PQ (s)	215	0.17	0.02	–	–	0.16	0.22	0.11	0.16	0.18	0.12	0.21
QRS (s)	214	0.09	0.01	–	–	0.09	0.13	0.06	0.09	0.10	0.07	0.11
QT (s)	215	0.40	0.03	–	–	0.40	0.49	0.32	0.38	0.42	0.35	0.46
QTc (s)	74	0.40	0.02	–	–	0.40	0.43	0.34	0.39	0.41	0.35	0.43
HR (bpm)	215	67.91	10.07	–	–	66	98	41	61	75	51	90
Age (years)	215	76.7	2.8	–	–	–	80	70	–	–	–	–

SD, Standard deviation; *CI-Up.*, 95% upper confidence limit; *CI-Lo.*, 95% lower confidence limit; *Med.*, median; *Max.*, maximum; *Min.*, minimum; *Lo.Q.*, lower quartile; *Up.Qt.*, upper quartile; *RR-Lo.L*, lower limit of reference range; *RR-Up.L*, upper limit of reference range.

6.3.1.2 Young Subjects

Table 144. ECG times: baseline, men aged 20–39 years (8:00–9:00 A.M.)

	n	Mean	SD	CI-Up.	CI-Lo.	Med.	Max.	Min.	Lo.Qt.	Up.Qt.	RR-Lo.L	RR-Up.L
RR (s)	547	1.013	0.151	1.026	1.000	1.00	1.46	0.64	0.90	1.12	0.73	1.30
P (s)	1030	0.099	0.012	0.100	0.098	0.10	0.14	0.06	0.09	0.10	0.08	0.12
PQ (s)	1638	0.159	0.021	0.160	0.158	0.16	0.28	0.10	0.14	0.17	0.12	0.20
QRS (s)	1638	0.094	0.011	0.094	0.093	0.09	0.14	0.05	0.09	0.10	0.07	0.11
QT (s)	1638	0.382	0.027	0.383	0.381	0.38	0.44	0.31	0.36	0.40	0.33	0.43
QTc (s)	601	0.385	0.023	0.387	0.383	0.39	0.44	0.31	0.37	0.40	0.34	0.43
HR (bpm)	1638	60.61	9.44	61.067	60.153	61	94.00	41.00	54	67	46	82
Age (years)	1638	27.91	4.45				39	20				

SD, Standard deviation; *CI-Up.*, 95% upper confidence limit; *CI-Lo.*, 95% lower confidence limit; *Med.*, median; *Max.*, maximum; *Min.*, minimum; *Lo.Q.*, lower quartile; *Up.Qt.*, upper quartile; *RR-Lo.L*, lower limit of reference range; *RR-Up.L*, upper limit of reference range.

Table 145. ECG times: baseline, men aged 20–29 and 30–39 years (8:00–9:00 A.M.)

n	Mean	SD	CI-Up.	CI-Lo.	Med.	Max.	Min.	Lo.Qt.	Up.Qt.	RR-Lo.L	RR-Up.L
20–29 years											
PQ (s)	1053	0.159	0.021	0.160	0.158	0.16	0.28	0.10	0.14	0.17	0.20
QRS (s)	1053	0.093	0.011	0.994	0.026	0.09	0.14	0.07	0.08	0.10	0.11
QT (s)	1053	0.382	0.027	0.384	0.380	0.38	0.47	0.32	0.36	0.40	0.43
Age (years)	1053	25.1	2.4	–	–	–	–	29	20	–	–
30–39 years											
PQ (s)	585	0.160	0.022	0.162	0.158	0.16	0.24	0.11	0.14	0.17	0.20
QRS (s)	585	0.094	0.011	0.095	0.093	0.09	0.16	0.05	0.08	0.10	0.12
QT (s)	585	0.383	0.030	0.385	0.381	0.38	0.47	0.31	0.36	0.40	0.44
Age (years)	585	33.0	2.4	–	–	–	–	39	30	–	–

SD, Standard deviation; *CI-Up.*, 95% upper confidence limit; *CI-Lo*, 95% lower confidence limit; *Med.*, median; *Max.*, maximum; *Min.*, minimum; *Lo.Q.*, lower quartile; *Up.Qt.*, upper quartile; *RR-Lo.L*, lower limit of reference range; *RR-Up.L*, upper limit of reference range.

6.3.2 Changes During Study Day

Table 146. ECG times: changes after 2 and 4 h, differences from baseline, men and women aged 50–80 years

n	Mean	SD	CI-Up.	CI-Lo.	Med.	Max.	Min.	RR-Lo.L	RR-Up.L	D$_{crit}$	
2 h											
RR (s)	130	0.05	0.11	0.066	0.028	0.06	0.32	−0.39	−0.21	0.26	0.20
PQ (s)	146	0.00	0.01	0.002	−0.002	0.00	0.03	−0.04	−0.02	0.02	0.02
QRS (s)	146	0.00	0.03	0.006	−0.003	0.00	0.33	−0.02	−0.02	0.02	0.02
QT (s)	146	0.01	0.02	0.010	0.004	0.01	0.05	−0.04	−0.03	0.04	0.04
HR (bpm)	146	−3.22	7.62	−1.984	−4.454	−4	24	−35	−16	17	15.9
Age (years)	146	67.7	6.1	–	–	–	76	51	–	–	–
4 h											
RR (s)	126	0.01	0.10	0.025	−0.010	0.01	0.32	−0.24	−0.21	0.20	0.20
PQ (s)	142	0.00	0.01	0.001	−0.002	0.00	0.03	−0.03	−0.02	0.02	0.02
QRS (s)	142	0.00	0.01	0.002	−0.001	0.00	0.02	−0.02	−0.02	0.02	0.02
QT (s)	142	0.00	0.02	0.004	−0.002	0.00	0.04	−0.05	−0.03	0.03	0.03
HR (bpm)	142	−0.88	6.48	0.185	−1.946	−1	15	−22	−14	11	13.5
Age (years)	142	66.4	6.3	–	–	–	76	51	–	–	–

SD, Standard deviation; *CI-Up.*, 95% upper confidence limit; *CI-Lo.*, 95% lower confidence limit; *Med.*, median; *Max.*, maximum; *Min.*, minimum; *RR-Lo.L*, lower limit of reference range; *RR-Up.L*, upper limit of reference range; *D$_{crit}$*, critical difference 0.05.

Table 147. ECG times: changes after 6 and 12 h, differences from baseline, men and women aged 50–80 years

	n	Mean	SD	CI-Up.	CI-Lo.	Med.	Max.	Min.	RR-Lo.L	RR-Up.L	D_{crit}
6 h											
RR (s)	199	−0.04	0.11	−0.027	−0.057	−0.03	0.28	−0.31	−0.27	0.19	0.22
PQ (s)	209	−0.001	0.01	0.001	−0.003	0.00	0.06	−0.07	−0.03	0.03	0.03
QRS (s)	209	0.001	0.01	0.002	0.000	0.00	0.02	−0.02	−0.01	0.02	0.02
QT (s)	209	−0.006	0.02	−0.004	−0.009	0.00	0.03	−0.06	−0.04	0.02	0.03
HR (bpm)	209	2.85	7.44	3.860	1.843	3.0	24	−31	−12	18	15.4
Age (years)	209	67.0	5.6	–	–	–	76	51	–	–	–
12 h											
RR (s)	69	−0.03	0.10	−0.011	−0.058	−0.03	0.26	−0.32	−0.27	0.15	0.21
PQ (s)	85	−0.004	0.01	−0.001	−0.007	0.00	0.02	−0.04	−0.03	0.02	0.03
QRS (s)	85	0.001	0.01	0.003	0.000	0.00	0.02	−0.02	−0.01	0.02	0.02
QT (s)	85	−0.01	0.02	−0.002	−0.010	−0.01	0.05	−0.04	−0.04	0.05	0.04
HR (bpm)	85	2.01	7.04	3.508	0.516	1.0	23	−24	−10	18	14.3
Age (years)	85	67.5	4.5	–	–	–	71	55	–	–	–

SD, Standard deviation; *CI-Up.*, 95% upper confidence limit; *CI-Lo.*, 95% lower confidence limit; *Med.*, median; *Max.*, maximum; *Min.*, minimum; *RR-Lo.L*, lower limit of reference range; *RR-Up.L*, upper limit of reference range.

6.3.3 Changes After Repeated Measurements

Table 148. ECG times: changes after 24 h, differences from baseline, men and women aged 50–80 years

	n	Mean	SD	CI-Up.	CI-Lo.	Med.	Max.	Min.	Lo.Qt.	Up.Qt.	RR-Lo.L	RR-Up.L	D_{crit}
RR (s)	180	-0.01	0.09	0.005	-0.022	-0.01	0.33	-0.33	-0.06	0.05	-0.17	0.19	0.19
PQ (s)	186	0.00	0.01	0.002	-0.002	0.00	0.06	-0.05	-0.01	0.01	-0.02	0.02	0.02
QRS (s)	186	0.00	0.01	0.001	-0.002	0.00	0.02	-0.02	0.00	0.00	-0.02	0.01	0.02
QT (s)	186	0.00	0.02	0.001	-0.004	0.00	0.05	-0.05	-0.01	0.01	-0.03	0.03	0.03
QTc (s)	180	0.00	0.02	0.003	-0.002	0.00	0.04	-0.07	-0.01	0.01	-0.03	0.03	0.04
HR (bpm)	186	0.51	7.14	1.536	-0.515	0	24	-33	-3	4	-12	15	14.3
Age (years)	186	67.4	5.5	–	–	76	51	–	–	–	–	–	–

SD, Standard deviation; CI-Up., 95% upper confidence limit; CI-Lo., 95% lower confidence limit; Med., median; Max., maximum; Min., minimum; Lo.Q., lower quartile; Up.Qt., upper quartile; RR-Lo.L, lower limit of reference range; RR-Up.L, upper limit of reference range; D_{crit} critical difference 0.05.

Table 149. ECG times: changes after 48 h, differences from baseline, men and women aged 50–80 years

	n	Mean	SD	CI-Up.	CI-Lo.	Med.	Max.	Min.	RR-Lo.L	RR-Up.L	D_{crit}
RR (s)	156	-0.01	0.10	0.002	-0.029	-0.01	0.36	-0.26	-0.22	0.15	0.19
PQ (s)	156	0.00	0.01	0.002	-0.002	0.00	0.06	-0.04	-0.03	0.03	0.03
QRS (s)	156	0.00	0.01	0.001	-0.002	0.00	0.02	-0.02	-0.02	0.01	0.02
QT (s)	156	0.00	0.02	0.000	-0.005	0.00	0.06	-0.04	-0.03	0.03	0.03
QTc (s)	156	0.00	0.02	0.003	-0.003	0.00	0.05	-0.04	-0.03	0.04	0.04
HR (bpm)	156	0.87	7.82	2.099	-0.355	1	21	-35	-14	15	16.1
Age (years)	156	67.7	5.5	–	–	76	59	–	–	–	–

SD, Standard deviation; CI-Up., 95% upper confidence limit; CI-Lo., 95% lower confidence limit; Med., median; Max., maximum; Min., minimum; RR-Lo.L, lower limit of reference range; RR-Up.L, upper limit of reference range; D_{crit} critical difference 0.05.

Table 150. ECG times: changes after 1 week, differences from baseline, men and women aged 50–80 years

	n	Mean	SD	CI-Up.	CI-Lo.	Med.	Max.	Min.	RR-Lo.L	RR-Up.L	D_{crit}
RR (s)	178	0.010	0.10	0.03	-0.01	0.005	0.35	-0.26	-0.21	0.21	0.21
PQ (s)	313	0.001	0.01	0.003	-0.001	0.000	0.04	-0.04	-0.03	0.03	0.03
QRS (s)	313	0.000	0.01	0.003	-0.001	0.000	0.03	-0.03	-0.02	0.02	0.02
QT (s)	313	-0.001	0.02	0.002	-0.003	0.000	0.08	-0.10	-0.04	0.04	0.05
QTc (s)	178	-0.003	0.02	0.000	-0.006	0.000	0.08	-0.06	-0.04	0.04	0.04
HR (bpm)	302	-0.51	7.55	0.34	-1.36	0	26	-34	-17	13	14.9
Age (years)	313	67.4	6.0	–	–	–	80	50	–	–	–

SD, Standard deviation; *CI-Up*, 95% upper confidence limit; *CI-Lo*, 95% lower confidence limit; *Med.*, median; *Max.*, maximum; *Min.*, minimum; *RR-Lo.L*, lower limit of reference range; *RR-Up.L*, upper limit of reference range; D_{crit} critical difference 0.05.

Table 151. ECG times: changes after 2 weeks, differences from baseline, men and women aged 50–80 years

	n	Mean	SD	CI-Up.	CI-Lo.	Med.	Max.	Min.	RR-Lo.L	RR-Up.L	D_{crit}
RR (s)	245	0.01	0.09	0.02	0.00	0.00	0.27	-0.32	-0.19	0.21	0.20
PQ (s)	280	0.001	0.014	0.002	-0.001	0.00	0.04	-0.05	-0.02	0.03	0.03
QRS (s)	280	0.000	0.010	0.001	-0.001	0.00	0.02	-0.03	-0.02	0.02	0.02
QT (s) (s)	280	0.001	0.019	0.003	-0.002	0.00	0.07	-0.05	-0.03	0.04	0.03
QTc (s)	202	-0.004	0.018	-0.001	-0.006	0.00	0.05	-0.06	-0.04	0.03	0.04
HR (bpm)	280	-1.14	7.69	-0.24	-2.04	-1	20	-43	-16	14	15.7
Age (years)	280	67.45	5.90	–	–	–	80	50	–	–	–

SD, Standard deviation; *CI-Up*, 95% upper confidence limit; *CI-Lo*, 95% lower confidence limit; *Med.*, median; *Max.*, maximum; *Min.*, minimum; *RR-Lo.L*, lower limit of reference range; *RR-Up.L*, upper limit of reference range; D_{crit} critical difference 0.05.

6.4 Ambulatory ECG Monitoring

6.4.1 Baseline Values

Table 152. Ambulatory ECG monitoring: baseline, men and women aged 50–80 years (start of registration between 8:00 and 9:00 A.M.)

	n	Mean	SD	CI-Up.	CI-Lo.	Med.	Max.	Min.	Lo.Qt.	Up.Qt.	RR-Lo.L	RR-Up.L
HR (bpm)	328	74.8	8.1	75.7	74.0	75	96	51	70	81	58	91
TEPS/24 h	328	13.4	22.9	15.9	10.9	6	182	0	2	16	0	80
BEPS/24 h	328	1.3	10.3	2.4	0.15	0	178	0	0	3	0	12
Pauses/24 h	328	6.8	74.7	14.9	−1.3	0	1236	0	0	4	0	11
SVE	328	58.3	208.0	80.9	35.8	8	2312	0	3	225	0	683
ISO	328	204.0	559.4	264.5	143.4	43	5031	0	14	232	1	1201
Age (years)	328	66.8	6.4	–	–	–	80	51	–	–	–	–

SD, Standard deviation; *CI-Up*, 95% upper confidence limit; *CI-Lo*, 95% lower confidence limit; *Med.*, median; *Max.*, maximum; *Min.*, minimum; *Lo.Q*, lower quartile; *Up.Qt.*, upper quartile; *RR-Lo.L*, lower limit of reference range; *RR-Up.L*, upper limit of reference range; *TEPS*, tachycardiac episodes; *BEPS*, bradycardiac episodes; *SVE*, supraventricular extrasystoles; *ISO*, isolated ventricular episodess.

Table 153. Ambulatory ECG monitoring: baseline, men aged 50–80 years (start of registration between 8:00 and 9:00 A.M.)

	n	Mean	SD	CI-Up.	CI-Lo.	Med.	Max.	Min.	Lo.Qt.	Up.Qt.	RR-Lo.L	RR-Up.L
HR (bpm)	172	74.8	8.2	76.1	73.6	75	93	51	69	81	59	91
TEPS/24 h	172	12.3	24.9	16.1	8.6	4	181	0	1	24	0	85
BEPS/24 h	172	0.64	2.55	1.02	0.26	0	21	0	0	3	0	11
Pauses/24 h	172	3.26	38.6	9.0	−2.5	0	506	0	0	4	0	7
SVE	172	50.8	173.5	76.7	24.9	7	1680	0	3	227	0	463
ISO	172	169.2	451.9	236.7	101.6	47	4462	0	12	220	0	1201
Age (years)	172	65.3	6.1	–	–	–	80	51	–	–	–	–

SD, Standard deviation; *CI-Up.*, 95% upper confidence limit; *CI-Lo.*, 95% lower confidence limit; *Med.*, median; *Max.*, maximum; *Min.*, minimum; *Lo.Q.*, lower quartile; *Up.Qt.*, upper quartile; *RR-Lo.L*, lower limit of reference range; *RR-Up.L*, upper limit of reference range; *TEPS*, tachycardiac episodes; *BEPS*, bradycardiac episodes; *SVE*, supraventricular extrasystoles; *ISO*, isolated ventricular episodess.

Table 154. Ambulatory ECG monitoring: baseline, women aged 50–80 years (start of registration between 8:00 and 9:00 A.M.)

	n	Mean	SD	CI-Up.	CI-Lo.	Med.	Max.	Min.	Lo.Qt.	Up.Qt.	RR-Lo.L	RR-Up.L
HR (bpm)	156	74.9	7.9	76.1	73.6	75	95	53	71	81	58	91
TEPS/24 h	156	14.6	20.5	17.8	11.4	9	116	0	2	18	0	78
BEPS/24 h	156	1.96	14.67	4.26	−0.34	0	177	0	0	0	0	16
Pauses/24 h	156	10.7	100.5	26.4	−5.12	6	1232	0	0	12	0	39
SVE	156	66.7	240.7	104.4	28.9	9	2315	0	3	225	0	683
ISO	156	242.4	657.3	345.5	139.2	143	5034	0	20	380	2	1609
Age (years)	156	67.5	6.7	–	–	–	80	51	–	–	–	–

SD, Standard deviation; *CI-Up.*, 95% upper confidence limit; *CI-Lo.*, 95% lower confidence limit; *Med.*, median; *Max.*, maximum; *Min.*, minimum; *Lo.Q.*, lower quartile; *Up.Qt.*, upper quartile; *RR-Lo.L*, lower limit of reference range; *RR-Up.L*, upper limit of reference range; *TEPS*, tachycardiac episodes; *BEPS*, bradycardiac episodes; *SVE*, supraventricular extrasystoles; *ISO*, isolated ventricular episodess.

6.4.2 Changes After 2–3 Weeks

Table 155. Ambulatory ECG monitoring: changes after 2–3 weeks, differences from baseine, men and women aged 50–80 years (start of registration between 8:00 and 9:00 A.M.)

	n	Mean	SD	CI-Up.	CI-Lo.	Med.	Max.	Min.	Lo.Qt.	Up.Qt.	RR-Lo.L	RR-Up.L	D_{crit}
HR (bpm)	168	-0.17	6.76	0.86	-1.19	0	19	-18	-4	4	-13	17	13.2
TEPS/24 h	168	1.38	23.9	5.0	-2.2	0	153	-109	-5	3	-49	55	42.1
BEPS/24 h	168	-1.3	14.9	0.9	-3.6	0	50	-175	-4	2	-13	5	8.8
Pauses/24 h	168	-2.9	24.5	0.8	-6.6	0	20	-245	-4	1	-10	11	9.4
SVE	168	3.1	188.2	31.6	-25.4	1	1371	-1077	-8	19	-360	270	332.6
ISO	168	-16.3	480.0	56.3	-88.8	-7	3543	-4162	-36	25	-592	529	520.8
Age (years)	168	66.0	6.1	–	–	–	78	54	–	–	–	–	–

SD, Standard deviation; *CI-Up.*, 95% upper confidence limit; *CI-Lo*, 95% lower confidence limit; *Med.*, median; *Max.*, maximum; *Min.*, minimum; *Lo.Q.*, lower quartile; *Up.Qt.*, upper quartile; *RR-Lo.L*, lower limit of reference range; *RR-Up.L*, upper limit of reference range; D_{crit} critical difference 0.05; *TEPS*, tachycardiac episodes; *BEPS*, bradycardiac episodes; *SVE*, supraventricular extrasystoles; *ISO*, isolated ventricular episodess.

6.5 Spirometry (FEV$_1$)

6.5.1 Baseline Values

6.5.1.1 Elderly Subjects

Table 156. FEV$_1$: baseline, men and women aged 50–80 years (8:00–9:00 A.M.)

	n	Mean	SD	CI-Up.	CI-Lo.	Med.	Max.	Min.	Lo.Qt.	Up.Qt.	RR-Lo.L	RR-Up.L
Men + women												
FEV$_1$ measured (l)	502	2.71	0.76	2.78	2.64	2.60	5.08	1.00	2.21	3.18	1.40	4.68
FEV$_1$ predicted (l)	502	2.68	0.59	2.73	2.62	2.68	3.93	1.21	2.21	3.12	1.64	3.74
Diff.(meas.–pred.;l)	502	0.03	0.57	0.08	−0.01	0.11	1.53	−1.84	−0.24	0.32	−1.37	1.18
Age (years)	502	66.9	6.7	–	–	–	80	51	–	–	–	–
Men												
FEV$_1$ measured (l)	240	3.05	0.78	3.15	2.96	2.92	5.08	1.00	2.48	3.48	1.96	4.84
FEV$_1$ predicted (l)	240	3.11	0.44	3.16	3.05	3.12	3.93	1.65	2.92	3.43	2.12	3.77
Diff.(meas.–pred.;l)	240	−0.05	0.71	0.04	−0.14	0.03	1.53	−1.84	−0.43	0.31	−1.60	1.33
Age (years)	240	66.9	6.8	–	–	–	80	53	–	–	–	–
Women												
FEV$_1$ measured (l)	262	2.40	0.59	2.47	2.33	2.36	3.99	1.12	1.96	2.81	1.36	3.52
FEV$_1$ predicted (l)	262	2.28	0.41	2.33	2.23	2.25	3.75	1.21	2.00	2.49	1.42	3.05
Diff.(meas.–pred.;l)	262	0.11	0.38	0.16	0.07	0.13	1.17	−0.94	−0.09	0.32	−0.72	0.97
Age (years)	262	66.9	6.6	–	–	–	80	51	–	–	–	–

SD, Standard deviation; CI-Up., 95% upper confidence limit; CI-Lo., 95% lower confidence limit; Med., median; Max., maximum; Min., minimum; Lo.Q., lower quartile; Up.Qt., upper quartile; RR-Lo.L, lower limit of reference range; RR-Up.L, upper limit of reference range.

Table 157. FEV1: baseline, men and women aged 50–59, 60–69, and 70–80 years (8:00–9:00 A.M.)

	n	Mean	SD	CI-Up.	CI-Lo.	Med.	Max.	Min.	Lo.Qt.	Up.Qt.	RR-Lo.L	RR-Up.L
50–59 years												
FEV$_1$ measured (l)	102	2.87	0.65	3.00	2.74	2.76	4.96	1.64	2.41	3.32	2.08	4.48
FEV$_1$ predicted (l)	102	2.88	0.53	2.98	2.78	2.90	3.86	1.97	2.43	3.36	2.19	3.74
Diff. (meas.–pred.; l)	102	–0.01	0.66	0.12	–0.14	0.13	1.22	–1.69	–0.34	0.45	–1.45	1.09
Age (years)	102	57.8	2.1	–	–	–	59	51	–	–	–	–
60–69 years												
FEV$_1$ measured (l)	268	2.73	0.79	2.83	2.64	2.68	5.08	1.00	2.20	3.17	1.52	4.76
FEV$_1$ predicted (l)	268	2.67	0.58	2.74	2.60	2.62	3.93	1.39	2.22	3.13	1.65	3.74
Diff. (meas.–pred.; l)	268	0.06	0.55	0.13	0.00	0.12	1.53	–1.84	1.11	0.32	–0.13	0.27
Age (years)	268	66.8	2.8	–	–	–	69	60	–	–	–	–
70–80 years												
FEV$_1$ measured (l)	132	2.55	0.77	2.68	2.42	2.40	4.68	1.12	2.12	3.12	1.32	4.32
FEV$_1$ predicted (l)	132	2.54	0.62	2.64	2.43	2.64	3.83	1.21	1.98	3.04	1.25	3.72
Diff. (meas.–pred.; l)	132	0.01	0.52	0.10	–0.08	0.08	1.23	–1.71	–0.24	0.27	–1.21	1.15
Age (years)	132	74.8	3.0	–	–	–	80	70	–	–	–	–

SD, Standard deviation; *CI-Up.*, 95% upper confidence limit; *CI-Lo*, 95% lower confidence limit; *Med.*, median; *Max.*, maximum; *Min.*, minimum; *Lo.Q.*, lower quartile; *Up.Qt.*, upper quartile; *RR-Lo.L*, lower limit of reference range; *RR-Up.L*, upper limit of reference range.

6.5.1.2 Young Subjects

Table 158. FEV1: baseline, men aged 20–39 years (8:00–9:00 A.M.)

	n	Mean	SD	CI-Up.	CI-Lo.	Med.	Max.	Min.	Lo.Qt.	Up.Qt.	RR-Lo.L	RR-Up.L
20–39 years												
FEV$_1$ measured (l)	433	4.57	0.47	4.61	4.52	4.56	5.92	3.48	4.28	4.88	3.68	5.56
FEV$_1$ predicted (l)	433	4.44	0.34	4.47	4.41	4.43	5.38	3.3	4.23	4.74	3.71	5.08
Diff (meas.–pred.; l)	433	0.13	0.37	0.16	0.09	0.10	0.86	−0.63	−0.18	0.40	−0.48	0.82
Age (years)	433	28.0	4.6	–	–	–	39	20	–	–	–	–
20–29 years												
FEV$_1$ measured (l)	294	4.61	0.47	4.67	4.56	4.60	5.92	3.58	4.32	4.88	3.76	5.64
FEV$_1$ predicted (l)	294	4.50	0.30	4.54	4.47	4.48	5.38	3.97	4.28	4.76	3.97	5.01
Diff (meas.–pred.; l)	294	0.11	0.38	0.15	0.07	0.06	0.86	−0.6	−0.2	0.4	−0.49	0.84
Age (years)	294	25.4	2.5	–	–	–	29	20	–	–	–	–
30–39 years												
FEV$_1$ measured (l)	139	4.48	0.46	4.55	4.40	4.52	5.28	3.48	4.20	4.84	3.56	5.20
FEV$_1$ predicted (l)	139	4.32	0.37	4.38	4.26	4.37	5.08	3.3	4.16	4.53	3.53	5.08
Diff (meas.–pred.; l)	139	0.16	0.35	0.21	0.10	0.15	0.86	−0.63	−0.14	0.41	−0.48	0.81
Age (years)	139	33.5	3.1	–	–	–	39	30	–	–	–	–

SD, Standard deviation; *CI-Up.*, 95% upper confidence limit; *CI-Lo*, 95% lower confidence limit; *Med.*, median; *Max.*, maximum; *Min*, minimum; *Lo.Q.*, lower quartile; *Up.Qt.*, upper quartile; *RR-Lo.L*, lower limit of reference range; *RR-Up.L*, upper limit of reference range.

6.5.2 Changes During Study Day and After 1 Week

Table 159. FEV1: changes after 4 h and 1 week, differences from baseline, men and women aged 50–80

	n	Mean	SD	CI-Up.	CI-Lo.	Med.	Max.	Min.	Lo.Qt.	Up.Qt.	RR-Lo.L	RR-Up.L	D_{crit}
After 4 h													
FEV$_1$	251	0.01	0.31	0.051	-0.025	-0.380	0.840	-2.68	-0.12	0.12	-0.60	0.56	0.60
Age (years)	251	65.5	5.7	–	–	–	76	51	–	–	–	–	–
After 1 week													
FEV$_1$	161	0.01	0.30	0.06	-0.04	0.04	1.04	-0.96	-0.16	0.16	-0.80	0.84	0.63
Age (years)	161	65.0	5.5	–	–	–	80	51	–	–	–	–	–

SD, Standard deviation; CI-Up., 95% upper confidence limit; CI-Lo., 95% lower confidence limit; Med., median; Max., maximum; Min., minimum; Lo.Q., lower quartile; Up.Qt., upper quartile; RR-Lo.L, lower limit of reference range; RR-Up.L, upper limit of reference range; D_{crit} critical difference 0.05.

6.6 Clinical Chemistry

6.6.1 Baseline Values

6.6.1.1 Elderly Subjects

Table 160. Clinical chemistry: fasting baseline, men and women aged 50–80 years, conventional units (7:00–9:00 A.M.)

	n	Mean	SD	CI-Up.	CI-Lo.	Med.	Max.	Min.	Lo.Qt.	Up.Qt.	RR-Lo.L	RR-Up.L
Alkaline phosphatase (U/l)	1138	106.09	28.49	107.74	104.43	103	292	38	85	124	55	169
AST (SGOT; U/l)	1142	9.22	2.87	9.38	9.05	9	29	3	7	10	6	18
ALT (SGPT; U/l)	1131	9.50	3.75	9.72	9.28	9	37	3	6	9	4	19
γ-GT (U/l)	1142	11.25	5.86	11.59	10.91	10	56	4	7	13	4	26
LDH (U/l)	829	173.11	46.46	176.27	169.95	164	396	77	143	188	114	303
Total bilirubin (mg/dl)	1095	0.52	0.20	0.53	0.51	0.48	1.25	0.13	0.38	0.62	0.24	1.07
Creatinine (mg/dl)	1095	0.76	0.14	0.77	0.75	0.75	1.32	0.44	0.66	0.86	0.52	1.08
Blood urea (BUN; mg/dl)	457	33.19	7.98	33.93	32.46	32.93	57.03	14.89	27.88	38.20	18.99	50.78
Uric acid (mg/dl)	1092	5.05	1.09	5.11	4.98	5.00	8.89	2.50	4.32	5.80	3.19	7.30
Total protein (g/dl)	995	7.19	0.45	7.22	7.16	7.20	9.90	5.80	6.91	7.53	6.31	8.09
Total cholesterol (mg/dl)	1034	241.88	34.90	244.01	239.76	242.98	303.01	120.30	217.80	281.86	173.06	298.09
Triglycerides (mg/dl)	994	127.56	53.13	130.86	124.26	119.96	273.01	40.85	86.21	158.18	55.83	254.92
Glucose fasting (mg/dl)	1081	100.69	12.56	101.44	99.94	99	146	61	92	108	79	129
Calcium (mmol/l)	372	2.34	0.12	2.36	2.33	2.35	2.56	1.97	2.26	2.44	2.08	2.55
Sodium (mmol/l)	1114	143.13	2.56	143.28	142.98	143.4	151.8	135.2	141.8	144.9	137.3	147.4
Potassium (mmol/l)	1137	4.44	0.36	4.46	4.42	4.38	5.91	3.43	4.19	4.63	3.83	5.30
Chloride (mmol/l)	952	104.39	3.19	104.59	104.18	104.4	110.9	92.1	102.3	106.6	97.7	110.3
Age (years)	1142	67.4	5.9	–	–	–	80	50	–	–	–	–

SD, Standard deviation; *CI-Up.*, 95% upper confidence limit; *CI-Lo.*, 95% lower confidence limit; *Med.*, median; *Max.*, maximum; *Min.*, minimum; *Lo.Q.*, lower quartile; *Up.Qt.*, upper quartile; *RR-Lo.L*, lower limit of reference range; *RR-Up.L*, upper limit of reference range.

Table 161. Clinical chemistry: fasting baseline, men and women aged 50–80 years, SI units (7:00–9:00 A.M.)

	n	Mean	SD	CI-Up.	CI-Lo.	Med.	Max.	Min.	Lo.Qt.	Up.Qt.	RR-Lo.L	RR-Up.L
Alkaline phosphatase (U/l)	1138	106.09	28.49	107.74	104.43	103	292	38	85	124	55	169
AST (SGOT; U/l)	1142	9.22	2.87	9.38	9.05	9	29	3	7	10	6	18
ALT (SGPT; U/l)	1131	9.50	3.75	9.72	9.28	9	37	3	6	9	4	19
γ-GT (U/l)	1142	11.25	5.86	11.59	10.91	10	56	4	7	13	4	26
LDH (U/l)	829	173.11	46.46	176.27	169.95	164	396	77	143	188	114	303
Total bilirubin (µmol/l)	1095	8.89	3.50	9.09	8.68	8.21	21.38	2.22	6.5	10.6	4.1	18.3
Creatinine (µmol/l)	1095	67.44	12.78	68.20	66.68	66.3	116.7	38.9	58.3	76.0	46.0	95.5
Blood urea (BUN; mmol/l)	457	5.53	1.33	5.65	5.41	5.48	9.50	2.48	4.64	6.36	3.16	8.45
Uric acid (µmol/l)	1092	300.20	64.57	304.03	296.37	297.43	528.82	148.71	256.98	345.01	189.76	434.24
Total protein (g/l)	995	71.92	4.53	72.20	71.64	72.1	98.9	58.0	69.1	75.3	63.1	80.9
Total cholesterol (mmol/l)	1034	6.24	0.90	6.30	6.19	6.27	7.82	3.10	5.62	7.27	4.46	7.69
Triglycerides (mmol/l)	994	1.45	0.61	1.49	1.42	1.37	3.11	0.47	0.98	1.80	0.64	2.91
Glucose fasting (mmol/l)	1081	5.59	0.70	5.63	5.55	5.49	8.10	3.39	5.11	5.99	4.38	7.16
Calcium (mmol/l)	372	2.34	0.12	2.36	2.33	2.35	2.56	1.97	2.26	2.44	2.08	2.55
Sodium (mmol/l)	1114	143.13	2.56	143.28	142.98	143.4	151.8	135.2	141.8	144.9	137.3	147.4
Potassium (mmol/l)	1137	4.44	0.36	4.46	4.42	4.38	5.91	3.43	4.19	4.63	3.83	5.30
Chloride (mmol/l)	952	104.39	3.19	104.59	104.18	104.4	110.9	92.1	102.3	106.6	97.7	110.3
Age (years)	1142	67.4	5.9	–	–	–	80	50	–	–	–	–

SD, Standard deviation; *CI-Up.*, 95% upper confidence limit; *CI-Lo*, 95% lower confidence limit; *Med.*, median; *Max.*, maximum; *Min.*, minimum; *Lo.Q.*, lower quartile; *Up.Qt.*, upper quartile; *RR-Lo.L*, lower limit of reference range; *RR-Up.L*, upper limit of reference range.

Table 162. Clinical chemistry: fasting baseline, men aged 50–80 years, conventional units (7:00–9:00 A.M.)

	n	Mean	SD	CI-Up.	CI-Lo.	Med.	Max.	Min.	Lo.Qt.	Up.Qt.	RR-Lo.L	RR-Up.L
Alkaline phosphatase (U/l)	539	105.21	29.85	107.73	102.69	102	292	44	84	123	54	171
AST (SGOT; U/l)	540	9.26	2.90	9.50	9.01	9	29	3	8	10	6	17
ALT (SGPT; U/l)	535	9.93	3.66	10.24	9.62	9	36	3	8	12	5	19
γ-GT (U/l)	540	13.27	6.18	13.79	12.75	12	50	4	9	16	5	29
LDH (U/l)	423	166.29	48.17	170.88	161.70	156	382	77	138	179	112	319
Total bilirubin (mg/dl)	517	0.56	0.21	0.58	0.55	0.52	1.25	0.18	0.42	0.68	0.25	1.12
Creatinine (mg/dl)	517	0.84	0.13	0.85	0.83	0.83	1.32	0.44	0.74	0.92	0.61	1.10
Blood urea (BUN; mg/dl)	226	32.24	7.38	33.20	31.28	32	51	15	27	37	19	48
Uric acid (mg/dl)	517	5.58	1.05	5.67	5.49	5.5	8.9	2.8	4.8	6.3	3.6	7.8
Total protein (g/dl)	459	7.22	0.44	7.26	7.18	7.2	9.6	5.8	6.9	7.5	6.3	8.1
Total cholesterol (mg/dl)	517	232.41	35.47	235.47	229.35	231	301	120	207	259	171	295
Triglycerides (mg/dl)	497	135.71	56.19	140.65	130.77	123	273	42	90	176	57	260
Glucose fasting (mg/dl)	511	101.76	12.34	102.83	100.69	100	146	72	94	109	79	133
Calcium (mmol/l)	180	2.35	0.12	2.37	2.33	2.36	2.56	1.97	2.28	2.44	2.12	2.54
Sodium (mmol/l)	524	143.19	2.65	143.41	142.96	143.45	151.8	135.2	141.6	145.0	137.5	147.6
Potassium (mmol/l)	535	4.45	0.37	4.48	4.42	4.40	5.87	3.40	4.19	4.67	3.79	5.30
Chloride (mmol/l)	445	104.12	3.28	104.43	103.82	104.0	110.9	92.0	102.2	106.5	97.6	110.5
Age (years)	540	66.1	5.4	–	–	–	80	50	–	–	–	–

SD, Standard deviation; *CI-Up.*, 95% upper confidence limit; *CI-Lo.*, 95% lower confidence limit; *Med.*, median; *Max.*, maximum; *Min.*, minimum; *Lo.Q.*, lower quartile; *Up.Qt.*, upper quartile; *RR-Lo.L*, lower limit of reference range; *RR-Up.L*, upper limit of reference range.

Table 163. Clinical chemistry: fasting baseline, men aged 50–80 years, SI units (7:00–9:00 A.M.)

	n	Mean	SD	CI-Up.	CI-Lo.	Med.	Max.	Min.	Lo.Qt.	Up.Qt.	RR-Lo.L	RR-Up.L
Alkaline phosphatase (U/l)	539	105.21	29.85	107.73	102.69	102	292	44	84	123	54	171
AST (SGOT; U/l)	540	9.26	2.90	9.50	9.01	9	29	3	8	10	6	17
ALT (SGPT; U/l)	535	9.93	3.66	10.24	9.62	9	36	3	8	12	5	19
γ-GT (U/l)	540	13.27	6.18	13.79	12.75	12	50	4	9	16	5	29
LDH (U/l)	423	166.29	48.17	170.88	161.70	156	382	77	138	179	112	319
Total bilirubin (μmol/l)	517	9.65	3.55	9.96	9.34	8.89	21.38	3.08	7.18	11.63	4.28	19.16
Creatinine (μmol/l)	517	73.96	11.60	74.96	72.95	73.37	116.69	38.90	65.42	81.33	53.92	97.24
Blood urea (BUN; mmol/l)	226	5.37	1.23	5.53	5.21	5.33	8.49	2.50	4.50	6.16	3.16	7.99
Uric acid (μmol/l)	517	331.98	62.75	337.39	326.57	327.17	529.42	166.56	285.53	374.76	214.15	463.98
Total protein (g/l)	459	72.20	4.39	72.60	71.80	72	96	58	69	75	63	81
Total cholesterol (mmol/l)	517	6.00	0.92	6.08	5.92	5.96	7.77	3.10	5.34	6.68	4.41	7.61
Triglycerides (mmol/l)	497	1.55	0.64	1.60	1.49	1.40	3.11	0.48	1.03	2.01	0.65	2.96
Glucose fasting (mmol/l)	511	5.65	0.68	5.71	5.59	5.55	8.10	4.00	5.22	6.05	4.38	7.38
Calcium (mmol/l)	180	2.35	0.12	2.37	2.33	2.36	2.56	1.97	2.28	2.44	2.12	2.54
Sodium (mmol/l)	524	143.19	2.65	143.41	142.96	143.45	151.8	135.2	141.6	145.0	137.5	147.6
Potassium (mmol/l)	535	4.45	0.37	4.48	4.42	4.40	5.87	3.40	4.19	4.67	3.79	5.30
Chloride (mmol/l)	445	104.12	3.28	104.43	103.82	104.00	110.90	92.00	102.20	106.50	97.60	110.50
Age (years)	540	66.1	5.4	–	–	–	80	50	–	–	–	–

SD, Standard deviation; *CI-Up.*, 95% upper confidence limit; *CI-Lo*, 95% lower confidence limit; *Med.*, median; *Max.*, maximum; *Min.*, minimum; *Lo.Q.*, lower quartile; *Up.Qt.*, upper quartile; *RR-Lo.L*, lower limit of reference range; *RR-Up.L*, upper limit of reference range.

Table 164. Clinical chemistry: fasting baseline, women aged 50–80 years, conventional units (7:00–9:00 A.M.)

	n	Mean	SD	CI-Up.	CI-Lo.	Med.	Max.	Min.	Lo.Qt.	Up.Qt.	RR-Lo.L	RR-Up.L
Alkaline phosphatase (U/l)	599	106.88	27.21	109.06	104.70	105	196	38	87	125	55	166
AST (SGOT; U/l)	602	9.18	2.84	9.41	8.96	9	26	5	7	10	5	18
ALT (SGPT; U/l)	596	9.12	3.79	9.42	8.81	8	37	3	7	11	4	18
γ-GT (U/l)	602	9.44	4.91	9.84	9.05	8	56	4	7	11	4	23
LDH (U/l)	406	180.22	43.55	184.46	175.98	173	396	81	152	196	122	295
Total bilirubin (mg/dl)	578	0.48	0.19	0.50	0.46	0.44	1.20	0.13	0.34	0.57	0.22	1.03
Creatinine (mg/dl)	578	0.70	0.12	0.71	0.69	0.68	1.21	0.48	0.61	0.77	0.52	0.98
Blood urea (BUN; mg/dl)	231	34.13	8.43	35.22	33.04	33	57	15	28	40	20	51
Uric acid (mg/dl)	575	4.57	0.87	4.64	4.50	4.5	7.0	2.5	4.0	5.1	3.0	6.4
Total protein (g/dl)	536	7.17	0.46	7.21	7.13	7.2	9.9	6.1	6.9	7.5	6.3	8.1
Total cholesterol (mg/dl)	517	251.36	31.63	254.08	248.63	255	303	146	229	278	189	299
Triglycerides (mg/dl)	497	119.41	48.58	123.68	115.14	110	266	41	82	149	56	244
Glucose fasting (mg/dl)	570	99.73	12.68	100.77	98.69	98	145	61	91	107	79	128
Calcium (mmol/l)	192	2.34	0.13	2.36	2.32	2.34	2.56	2.03	2.24	2.45	2.07	2.55
Sodium (mmol/l)	590	143.07	2.49	143.27	142.87	143.3	148.4	135.2	141.9	144.8	137.0	147.0
Potassium (mmol/l)	602	4.42	0.35	4.45	4.40	4.37	5.90	3.60	4.20	4.63	3.87	5.24
Chloride (mmol/l)	507	104.62	3.09	104.89	104.35	104.8	110.8	95.0	102.5	106.7	98.0	110.1
Age (years)	602	66.4	5.5	–	–	–	80	54	–	–	–	–

SD, Standard deviation; *CI-Up.*, 95% upper confidence limit; *CI-Lo.*, 95% lower confidence limit; *Med.*, median; *Max.*, maximum; *Min.*, minimum; *Lo.Q.*, lower quartile; *Up.Qt.*, upper quartile; *RR-Lo.L*, lower limit of reference range; *RR-Up.L*, upper limit of reference range.

Table 165. Clinical chemistry: fasting baseline, women aged 50–80 years, SI units (7:00–9:00 A.M.)

	n	Mean	SD	CI-Up.	CI-Lo.	Med.	Max.	Min.	Lo.Qt.	Up.Qt.	RR-Lo.L	RR-Up.L
Alkaline phosphatase (U/l)	599	106.88	27.21	109.06	104.70	105	196	38	87	125	55	166
AST (SGOT; U/l)	602	9.18	2.84	9.41	8.96	9	26	5	7	10	5	18
ALT (SGPT; U/l)	596	9.12	3.79	9.42	8.81	8	37	3	7	11	4	18
γ-GT (U/l)	602	9.44	4.91	9.84	9.05	8	56	4	7	11	4	23
LDH (U/l)	406	180.22	43.55	184.46	175.98	173	396	81	152	196	122	295
Total bilirubin (μmol/l)	578	8.21	3.30	8.47	7.94	7.53	20.52	2.22	5.82	9.75	3.76	17.62
Creatinine (μmol/l)	578	61.61	10.82	62.50	60.73	60.11	106.96	42.43	53.92	68.07	45.97	86.63
Blood urea (BUN; mmol/l)	231	5.68	1.40	5.86	5.50	5.49	9.49	2.50	4.66	6.66	3.33	8.49
Uric acid (μmol/l)	575	271.62	51.54	275.84	267.41	267.7	416.4	148.7	237.9	303.4	178.5	380.70
Total protein (g/l)	536	71.68	4.64	72.08	71.29	72	99	61	69	75	63	81
Total cholesterol (mmol/l)	517	6.48	0.82	6.56	6.41	6.58	7.82	3.77	5.91	7.17	4.88	7.71
Triglycerides (mmol/l)	497	1.36	0.55	1.41	1.31	1.25	3.03	0.47	0.93	1.70	0.64	2.78
Glucose fasting (mmol/l)	570	5.54	0.70	5.59	5.48	5.44	8.05	3.39	5.05	5.94	4.38	7.10
Calcium (mmol/l)	192	2.34	0.13	2.36	2.32	2.34	2.56	2.03	2.24	2.45	2.07	2.55
Sodium (mmol/l)	590	143.07	2.49	143.27	142.87	143.3	148.4	135.2	141.9	144.8	137.0	147.0
Potassium (mmol/l)	602	4.42	0.35	4.45	4.40	4.37	5.90	3.60	4.20	4.63	3.87	5.24
Chloride (mmol/l)	507	104.62	3.09	104.89	104.35	104.8	110.8	95.0	102.5	106.7	98.0	110.1
Age (years)	602	68.4	5.5	–	–	–	80	54	–	–	–	–

SD, Standard deviation; *CI-Up.*, 95% upper confidence limit; *CI-Lo*, 95% lower confidence limit; *Med.*, median; *Max.*, maximum; *Min.*, minimum; *Lo.Q.*, lower quartile; *Up.Qt.*, upper quartile; *RR-Lo.L*, lower limit of reference range; *RR-Up.L*, upper limit of reference range.

Table 166. Clinical chemistry: fasting baseline, men and women aged 50–59 years, conventional units (7:00–9:00 A.M.)

	n	Mean	SD	CI-Up.	CI-Lo.	Med.	Max.	Min.	Lo.Qt.	Up.Qt.	RR-Lo.L	RR-Up.L
Alkaline phosphatase (U/l)	188	105.31	28.34	109.36	101.26	103	189.00	48	85.00	122.00	57	167
AST (SGOT; U/l)	190	9.41	3.26	9.87	8.95	9	29.00	5	8.00	10.00	5	20
ALT (SGPT; U/l)	189	9.79	3.63	10.31	9.28	9	25.00	3	7.00	12.00	5	18
γ-GT (U/l)	190	11.69	6.29	12.58	10.79	11	50.00	4	8.00	14.00	5	27
LDH (U/l)	162	173.59	46.89	180.81	166.37	162	382.00	85	146.00	189.00	119	309
Total bilirubin (mg/dl)	183	0.53	0.20	0.55	0.50	0.49	1.23	0.11	0.38	0.62	0.24	1.05
Creatinine (mg/dl)	183	0.75	0.14	0.77	0.73	0.73	1.17	0.35	0.65	0.85	0.52	1.06
Uric acid (mg/dl)	183	5.07	1.00	5.21	4.92	5.2	7.60	3.1	4.40	5.70	3.3	7.1
Total protein (g/dl)	156	7.16	0.41	7.23	7.10	7.15	8.20	6.0	6.90	7.40	6.4	8.0
Total cholesterol (mg/dl)	174	243.22	35.32	248.47	237.98	243.2	301.0	154.1	218.9	275.2	172	296
Triglycerides (mg/dl)	170	137.18	55.99	145.59	128.76	131.5	261.0	43.2	91.1	176.2	54	257
Glucose fasting (mg/dl)	183	101.50	13.16	103.41	99.60	99.3	145.0	72.3	92.0	108.1	80	134
Sodium (mmol/l)	179	142.94	2.85	143.36	142.53	143.4	151.8	135.4	141.3	145.0	136.	147.2
Potassium (mmol/l)	188	4.44	0.36	4.49	4.39	4.39	5.90	4.01	4.20	4.63	3.80	5.38
Chloride (mmol/l)	173	104.36	3.20	104.83	103.88	104.2	110.9	92.1	102.6	106.4	97.3	109.9
Age (years)	190	57.5	1.6	–	–	–	59	50	–	–	–	–

SD, Standard deviation; *CI-Up.*, 95% upper confidence limit; *CI-Lo*, 95% lower confidence limit; *Med*, median; *Max*, maximum; *Min*, minimum; *Lo.Q*, lower quartile; *Up.Qt*, upper quartile; *RR-Lo.L*, lower limit of reference range; *RR-Up.L*, upper limit of reference range.

Table 167. Clinical chemistry: fasting baseline, men and women aged 50–59 years, SI units (7:00–9:00 A.M.)

	n	Mean	SD	CI-Up.	CI-Lo.	Med.	Max.	Min.	Lo.Qt.	Up.Qt.	RR-Lo.L	RR-Up.L
Alkaline phosphatase (U/l)	188	105.31	28.34	109.36	101.26	103	189	48	85	122	57	167
AST (SGOT; U/l)	190	9.41	3.26	9.87	8.95	9	29	5	8	10	5	20
ALT (SGPT; U/l)	189	9.79	3.63	10.31	9.28	9	25	3	7	12	5	18
γ-GT (U/l)	190	11.69	6.29	12.58	10.79	11	50	4	8	14	5	27
LDH (U/l)	162	173.59	46.89	180.81	166.37	162	382	85	146	189	119	309
Total bilirubin (µmol/l)	183	8.99	3.47	9.49	8.49	8.38	21.04	3.42	6.50	10.60	4.10	17.96
Creatinine (µmol/l)	183	66.45	12.41	68.25	64.66	64.53	103.43	44.20	57.46	75.14	45.97	93.70
Uric acid (µmol/l)	183	301.52	59.49	310.14	292.90	297.43	452.09	148.71	261.73	339.06	196.30	422.34
Total protein (g/l)	156	71.63	4.14	72.28	70.98	71.50	82	62	69	74	64	80
Total cholesterol (mmol/l)	174	6.28	0.91	6.41	6.14	6.27	7.77	3.97	5.65	7.10	4.44	7.64
Triglycerides (mmol/l)	170	1.56	0.64	1.66	1.47	1.50	2.98	0.49	1.04	2.01	0.62	2.93
Glucose fasting (mmol/l)	183	5.63	0.73	5.74	5.53	5.49	8.05	4.00	5.11	5.99	4.44	7.44
Sodium (mmol/l)	179	142.94	2.85	143.36	142.53	143.4	151.8	135.2	141.3	145.0	136.0	147.2
Potassium (mmol/l)	188	4.44	0.36	4.49	4.39	4.39	5.90	3.63	4.20	4.63	3.80	5.38
Chloride (mmol/l)	173	104.36	3.20	104.83	103.88	104.2	110.9	92.0	102.6	106.4	97.3	109.9
Age (years)	190	57.5	1.6	–	–	–	59	50	–	–	–	–

SD, Standard deviation; *CI-Up.,* 95% upper confidence limit; *CI-Lo.,* 95% lower confidence limit; *Med.,* median; *Max.,* maximum; *Min.,* minimum; *Lo.Q.,* lower quartile; *Up.Qt.,* upper quartile; *RR-Lo.L,* lower limit of reference range; *RR-Up.L,* upper limit of reference range.

Table 168. Clinical chemistry: fasting baseline, men and women aged 60–69 years, conventional units (7:00–9:00 A.M.)

	n	Mean	SD	CI-Up.	CI-Lo.	Med.	Max.	Min.	Lo.Qt.	Up.Qt.	RR-Lo.L	RR-Up.L
Alkaline phosphatase (U/l)	713	107.25	28.99	109.38	105.12	105	292	40	86	119	56	171
AST (SGOT; U/l)	715	9.29	2.80	9.49	9.08	9	25	3	8	10	6	18
ALT (SGPT; U/l)	706	9.55	3.88	9.84	9.27	9	37	3	7	11	4	19
γ-GT (U/l)	715	11.28	5.75	11.70	10.86	10	56	4	7	13	5	26
LDH (U/l)	516	174.30	46.95	178.35	170.25	166	396	77	145	189	116	350
Total bilirubin (mg/dl)	686	0.53	0.21	0.54	0.51	0.48	1.25	0.13	0.38	0.64	0.23	1.17
Creatinine (mg/dl)	686	0.76	0.14	0.77	0.75	0.75	1.32	0.44	0.66	0.86	0.52	1.09
Blood urea (BUN; mg/dl)	296	33.30	7.89	34.20	32.40	32	56	15	28	39	20	51
Uric acid (mg/dl)	685	5.04	1.08	5.12	4.96	5.0	8.9	2.8	4.3	5.8	3.2	7.4
Total protein (g/dl)	622	7.21	0.46	7.25	7.18	7.2	8.9	6.0	6.9	7.5	6.3	8.1
Total cholesterol (mg/dl)	652	242.23	34.74	244.89	239.56	244	302	124	218	271	174	298
Triglycerides (mg/dl)	626	125.59	53.65	129.80	121.39	112	273	41	85	156	57	259
Glucose fasting (mg/dl)	675	100.25	12.07	101.16	99.34	99	145	62	93	108	79	128
Calcium (mmol/l)	240	2.34	0.13	2.35	2.32	2.34	2.56	2.03	2.25	2.45	2.09	2.55
Sodium (mmol/l)	705	143.07	2.50	143.25	142.89	143.2	150.0	135.2	141.8	144.8	137.5	147.6
Potassium (mmol/l)	712	4.45	0.37	4.47	4.42	4.40	5.87	3.40	4.19	4.66	3.87	5.30
Chloride (mmol/l)	593	104.42	3.15	104.67	104.17	104.4	110.9	95.0	102.3	106.7	98.0	110.2
Age (years)	715	66.0	2.3	–	–	–	69	60	–	–	–	–

SD, Standard deviation; CI-Up., 95% upper confidence limit; CI-Lo., 95% lower confidence limit; Med., median; Max., maximum; Min., minimum; Lo.Q, lower quartile; Up.Qt., upper quartile; RR-Lo.L, lower limit of reference range; RR-Up.L, upper limit of reference range.

Table 169. Clinical chemistry: fasting baseline, men and women aged 60–69 years, SI units (7:00–9:00 A.M.)

	n	Mean	SD	CI-Up.	CI-Lo.	Med.	Max.	Min.	Lo.Qt.	Up.Qt.	RR-Lo.L	RR-Up.L
Alkaline phosphatase (U/l)	713	107.25	28.99	109.38	105.12	105	292	40	86	119	56	171
AST (SGOT; U/l)	715	9.29	2.80	9.49	9.08	9	25	3	8	10	6	18
ALT (SGPT; U/l)	706	9.55	3.88	9.84	9.27	9	37	3	7	11	4	19
γ-GT (U/l)	715	11.28	5.75	11.70	10.86	10	56	4	7	13	5	26
LDH (U/l)	516	174.30	46.95	178.35	170.25	166	396	77	145	189	116	350
Total bilirubin (μmol/l)	686	8.99	3.66	9.27	8.72	8.21	21.38	2.22	6.50	10.95	3.93	20.01
Creatinine (μmol/l)	686	67.35	12.78	68.31	66.40	66.30	116.69	38.90	58.34	76.02	45.97	96.36
Blood urea (BUN; mmol/l)	296	5.54	1.31	5.69	5.39	5.33	9.32	2.50	4.66	6.49	3.33	8.49
Uric acid (μmol/l)	685	300.04	64.36	304.86	295.22	297.43	529.42	166.56	255.79	345.01	190.35	440.19
Total protein (g/l)	622	72.13	4.60	72.49	71.77	72	89	60	69	75	63	81
Total cholesterol (mmol/l)	652	6.25	0.90	6.32	6.18	6.30	7.79	3.20	5.62	6.99	4.49	7.69
Triglycerides (mmol/l)	626	1.43	0.61	1.48	1.38	1.28	3.11	0.47	0.97	1.78	0.65	2.95
Glucose fasting (mmol/l)	675	5.56	0.67	5.61	5.51	5.49	8.05	3.44	5.16	5.99	4.38	7.10
Calcium (mmol/l)	240	2.34	0.13	2.35	2.32	2.34	2.56	2.03	2.25	2.45	2.09	2.55
Sodium (mmol/l)	705	143.07	2.50	143.25	142.89	143.2	150.0	135.2	141.8	144.8	137.5	147.6
Potassium (mmol/l)	712	4.45	0.37	4.47	4.42	4.40	5.87	3.40	4.19	4.66	3.87	5.30
Chloride (mmol/l)	593	104.42	3.15	104.67	104.17	104.4	110.9	95.0	102.3	106.7	98.0	110.2
Age (years)	715	66.03	2.3	–	–	–	69	60	–	–	–	–

SD, Standard deviation; *CI-Up.*, 95% upper confidence limit; *CI-Lo*, 95% lower confidence limit; *Med.*, median; *Max.*, maximum; *Min.*, minimum; *Lo.Q.*, lower quartile; *Up.Qt.*, upper quartile; *RR-Lo.L*, lower limit of reference range; *RR-Up.L*, upper limit of reference range.

Table 170. Clinical chemistry: fasting baseline, men and women aged 70–80 years, conventional units (7:00–9:00 A.M.)

	n	Mean	SD	CI-Up.	CI-Lo.	Med.	Max.	Min.	Lo.Qt.	Up.Qt.	RR-Lo.L	RR-Up.L
Alkaline phosphatase (U/l)	237	103.20	26.95	106.63	99.77	103	189	38	83	120	55	173
AST (SGOT; U/l)	237	8.85	2.71	9.19	8.50	8	23	5	7	10	6	19
ALT (SGPT; U/l)	236	9.11	3.42	9.55	8.68	8	23	3	7	11	5	21
γ-GT (U/l)	237	10.81	5.85	11.56	10.07	9	47	4	7	13	4	31
LDH (U/l)	151	168.54	44.30	175.60	161.47	160	380	81	142	184	118	380
Total bilirubin (mg/dl)	226	0.50	0.17	0.52	0.47	0.48	1.18	0.23	0.38	0.58	0.26	1.04
Creatinine (mg/dl)	226	0.78	0.15	0.79	0.76	0.78	1.20	0.44	0.67	0.89	0.54	1.10
Blood urea (BUN; mg/dl)	103	34.22	8.13	35.79	32.65	33	57	15	30	41	20	57
Uric acid (mg/dl)	224	5.04	1.16	5.19	4.88	4.9	8.7	2.7	4.2	5.9	3.2	8.2
Total protein (g/dl)	217	7.15	0.46	7.21	7.09	7.2	9.4	5.8	6.9	7.5	6.3	8.1
Total cholesterol (mg/dl)	208	239.69	35.11	244.46	234.92	238	303	120	218	268	175	299
Triglycerides (mg/dl)	198	125.53	48.07	132.23	118.83	117	271	42	91	156	60	258
Glucose fasting (mg/dl)	223	101.35	13.46	103.11	99.58	99	146	61	93	110	81	135
Sodium (mmol/l)	230	143.44	2.50	143.77	143.12	143.6	151.0	135.9	142.3	145.2	137.8	147.9
Potassium (mmol/l)	237	4.41	0.35	4.46	4.37	4.35	5.81	3.60	4.20	4.62	3.90	5.26
Chloride (mmol/l)	186	104.31	3.33	104.79	103.83	104.3	110.9	94.5	102.2	106.8	98.0	110.8
Age (years)	237	73.9	2.8	–	–	–	80	70	–	–	–	–

SD, Standard deviation; *CI-Up*, 95% upper confidence limit; *CI-Lo*, 95% lower confidence limit; *Med*, median; *Max.*, maximum; *Min.*, minimum; *Lo.Q*, lower quartile; *Up.Qt*, upper quartile; *RR-Lo.L*, lower limit of reference range; *RR-Up.L*, upper limit of reference range.

Table 171. Clinical chemistry: fasting baseline, men and women aged 70–80 years, SI units (7:00–9:00 A.M.)

	n	Mean	SD	CI-Up.	CI-Lo.	Med.	Max.	Min.	Lo.Qt.	Up.Qt.	RR-Lo.L	RR-Up.L
Alkaline phosphatase (U/l)	237	103.20	26.95	106.63	99.77	103	189	38	83	120	55	173
AST (SGOT; U/l)	237	8.85	2.71	9.19	8.50	8	23	5	7	10	6	19
ALT (SGPT; U/l)	236	9.11	3.42	9.55	8.68	8	23	3	7	11	5	21
γ-GT (U/l)	237	10.81	5.85	11.56	10.07	9	47	4	7	13	4	31
LDH (U/l)	151	168.54	44.30	175.60	161.47	160	380	81	142	184	118	380
Total bilirubin (μmol/l)	226	8.49	2.94	8.87	8.10	8.12	20.18	3.93	6.50	9.92	4.45	17.79
Creatinine (μmol/l)	226	68.51	13.05	70.21	66.81	68.51	106.08	38.90	59.23	78.68	47.74	97.24
Blood urea (BUN; mmol/l)	103	5.70	1.35	5.96	5.44	5.49	9.49	2.50	5.00	6.83	3.33	9.49
Uric acid (μmol/l)	224	299.60	69.27	308.67	290.53	291.48	517.52	160.61	249.84	350.96	190.35	487.78
Total protein (g/l)	217	71.53	4.59	72.15	70.92	72	94	58	69	75	63	81
Total cholesterol (mmol/l)	208	6.18	0.91	6.31	6.06	6.14	7.82	3.10	5.62	6.91	4.52	7.71
Triglycerides (mmol/l)	198	1.43	0.55	1.51	1.35	1.33	3.09	0.48	1.04	1.78	0.68	2.94
Glucose fasting (mmol/l)	223	5.62	0.75	5.72	5.53	5.49	8.10	3.39	5.16	6.11	4.50	7.49
Sodium (mmol/l)	230	143.44	2.50	143.77	143.12	143.6	151.0	135.9	142.3	145.2	137.8	147.9
Potassium (mmol/l)	237	4.41	0.35	4.46	4.37	4.35	5.81	3.60	4.20	4.62	3.90	5.26
Chloride (mmol/l)	186	104.31	3.33	104.79	103.83	104.3	110.9	94.5	102.2	106.8	98.0	110.8
Age (years)	237	73.9	2.8	–	–	–	80	70	–	–	–	–

SD, Standard deviation; CI-Up., 95% upper confidence limit; CI-Lo., 95% lower confidence limit; Med., median; Max., maximum; Min., minimum; Lo.Q., lower quartile; Up.Qt., upper quartile; RR-Lo.L, lower limit of reference range; RR-Up.L, upper limit of reference range.

6.6.1.2 Young Subjects

Table 172. Clinical chemistry: fasting baseline, men aged 20–39 years, conventional units (7:00–9:00 A.M.)

	n	Mean	SD	CI-Up.	CI-Lo.	Med.	Max.	Min.	Lo.Qt.	Up.Qt.	RR-Lo.L	RR-Up.L
Alkaline phosphatase (U/l)	1485	95.21	23.21	96.39	94.03	92	188	31	78	110	58	146
AST (SGOT; U/l)	1334	9.55	3.31	9.73	9.37	9	49	4	8	11	6	17
ALT (SGPT; U/l)	1333	10.25	5.11	10.52	9.98	9	61	3	7	12	5	21
γ-GT (U/l)	1333	10.27	4.84	10.53	10.01	9	79	2	7	12	5	24
LDH (U/l)	1346	154.20	43.19	156.51	151.90	146	411	15	128	169	97	260
Total bilirubin (mg/dl)	1156	0.51	0.24	0.53	0.50	0.46	1.6	0.1	0.33	0.66	0.2	1.1
Creatinine (mg/dl)	1499	0.83	0.12	0.84	0.83	0.82	1.24	0.39	0.76	0.89	0.65	1.11
Blood urea (BUN; mg/dl)	1177	29.60	8.11	30.06	29.14	29	83	10	24	34	16	47
Uric acid (mg/dl)	1064	5.33	1.01	5.39	5.27	5.3	11.6	2.60	4.7	6.2	3.4	7.2
Total protein (g/dl)	1489	7.25	0.53	7.28	7.22	7.2	9.6	5.0	7.0	7.6	6.1	8.3
Total cholesterol (mg/dl)	1449	188.22	34.07	189.98	186.47	187	420	98	166	209	124	256
Triglycerides (mg/dl)	1105	114.18	57.02	117.54	110.81	101	451	24	73	140	45	265
Glucose fasting (mg/dl)	1458	91.32	10.43	91.86	90.79	91	139	54	85	97	71	114
Calcium (mmol/l)	839	2.35	0.12	2.35	2.34	2.36	2.6	1.82	2.29	2.42	2.04	2.55
Sodium (mmol/l)	1375	143.62	2.85	143.77	143.47	143.7	157.0	135.1	142.0	145.2	138.1	149.0
Potassium (mmol/l)	1480	4.36	0.34	4.38	4.35	4.35	6.63	3.44	4.12	4.59	3.73	5.10
Chloride (mmol/l)	1296	105.79	4.71	106.04	105.53	105.4	127.1	89.3	102.7	108.2	97.8	117.0
Age (years)	1499	27.2	3.8	–	–	–	39	20	–	–	–	–

SD, Standard deviation; *CI-Up.*, 95% upper confidence limit; *CI-Lo*, 95% lower confidence limit; *Med.*, median; *Max.*, maximum; *Min.*, minimum; *Lo.Q.*, lower quartile; *Up.Qt.*, upper quartile; *RR-Lo.L*, lower limit of reference range; *RR-Up.L*, upper limit of reference range.

Table 173. Clinical chemistry: fasting baseline, men aged 20–39 years, SI units (7:00–9:00 A.M.)

	n	Mean	SD	CI-Up.	CI-Lo.	Med.	Max.	Min.	Lo.Qt.	Up.Qt.	RR-Lo.L	RR-Up.L
Alkaline phosphatase (U/l)	1485	95.21	23.21	96.39	94.03	92	188	31	78	110	58	146
AST (SGOT; U/l)	1334	9.55	3.31	9.73	9.37	9	49	4	8	11	6	17
ALT (SGPT; U/l)	1333	10.25	5.11	10.52	9.98	9	61	3	7	12	5	21
γ-GT (U/l)	1333	10.27	4.84	10.53	10.01	9	79	2	7	12	5	24
LDH (U/l)	1346	154.20	43.19	156.51	151.90	146	411	15	128	169	97	260
Total bilirubin (µmol/l)	1156	8.80	4.17	9.04	8.56	7.87	27.37	1.71	5.64	11.29	3.42	18.81
Creatinine (µmol/l)	1499	73.70	10.54	74.23	73.16	72.49	109.62	34.48	67.18	78.68	57.46	98.12
Blood urea (BUN; mmol/l)	1177	4.93	1.35	5.01	4.85	4.83	14.99	1.67	4.00	5.66	2.66	7.83
Uric acid (µmol/l)	1064	316.98	60.35	320.44	313.20	315.27	690.03	154.66	279.58	356.91	202.25	428.29
Total protein (g/l)	1489	72.52	5.30	72.79	72.25	72	96	50.2	71.3	76.1	61.0	83.1
Total cholesterol (mmol/l)	1449	4.86	0.88	4.90	4.81	4.82	10.84	2.53	4.28	5.39	3.20	6.60
Triglycerides (mmol/l)	1105	1.30	0.65	1.34	1.26	1.15	5.14	0.27	0.83	1.60	0.51	3.02
Glucose fasting (mmol/l)	1458	5.07	0.58	5.10	5.04	5.05	7.71	3.00	4.72	5.38	3.94	6.33
Calcium (mmol/l)	839	2.35	0.12	2.35	2.34	2.36	2.6	1.82	2.29	2.42	2.04	2.55
Sodium (mmol/l)	1375	143.62	2.85	143.77	143.47	143.7	157.2	135.1	142.0	145.2	138.1	149.0
Potassium (mmol/l)	1480	4.36	0.34	4.38	4.35	4.35	6.63	3.44	4.12	4.59	3.73	5.1
Chloride (mmol/l)	1296	105.79	4.71	106.04	105.53	105.4	127.1	89.3	102.7	108.0	97.8	117.0
Age (years)	1499	27.2	3.8	-	-	-	39	20	-	-	-	-

SD, Standard deviation; *CI-Up.*, 95% upper confidence limit; *CI-Lo*, 95% lower confidence limit; *Med.*, median; *Max.*, maximum; *Min.*, minimum; *Lo.Q.*, lower quartile; *Up.Qt.*, upper quartile; *RR-Lo.L*, lower limit of reference range; *RR-Up.L*, upper limit of reference range.

Table 174. Clinical chemistry: fasting baseline, men aged 20–29 years, conventional units (7:00–9:00 A.M.)

	n	Mean	SD	CI-Up.	CI-Lo.	Med.	Max.	Min.	Lo.Qt.	Up.Qt.	RR-Lo.L	RR-Up.L
Alkaline phosphatase (U/l)	1159	95.11	22.73	96.42	93.80	92	172	31	78	111	57	143
AST (SGOT; U/l)	1049	9.69	3.47	9.90	9.48	9	49	4	8	11	6	18
ALT (SGPT; U/l)	1048	10.27	5.08	10.58	9.96	9	61	3	7	12	5	22
γ-GT (U/l)	1048	10.26	5.06	10.57	9.96	9	79	2	7	12	5	25
LDH (U/l)	1068	156.04	46.02	158.80	153.28	147	411	15	129	173	93	265
Total bilirubin (mg/dl)	923	0.52	0.25	0.54	0.50	0.48	1.60	0.10	0.32	0.68	0.20	1.10
Creatinine (mg/dl)	1171	0.84	0.12	0.84	0.83	0.82	1.24	0.39	0.76	0.90	0.66	1.12
Blood urea (BUN; mg/dl)	951	29.12	7.81	29.62	28.62	29	58	10	24	34	15	46
Uric acid (mg/dl)	774	5.33	1.01	5.40	5.26	5.3	11.6	2.5	4.6	6.0	3.4	7.2
Total protein (g/dl)	1164	7.25	0.55	7.28	7.21	7.1	9.3	5.0	7.0	7.6	6.0	8.3
Total cholesterol (mg/dl)	1141	184.56	34.58	186.57	182.55	183	420	98	163	205	122	254
Triglycerides (mg/dl)	888	115.19	59.38	119.10	111.28	99	451	24	73	144	44	276
Glucose fasting (mg/dl)	1146	90.94	10.67	91.56	90.32	90	139	54	85	97	70	114
Calcium (mmol/l)	611	2.34	0.13	2.35	2.33	2.36	2.60	1.82	2.28	2.43	2.04	2.56
Sodium (mmol/l)	1076	143.69	2.95	143.87	143.52	143.7	157.0	135.1	142.0	145.5	138.1	149.2
Potassium (mmol/l)	1161	4.36	0.34	4.38	4.34	4.35	5.98	3.44	4.10	4.59	3.72	5.10
Chloride (mmol/l)	1027	106.03	4.89	106.33	105.73	105.9	127.0	89.0	102.9	108.8	97.8	118.0
Age (years)	1171	25.7	2.4	–	–	–	29	20	–	–	–	–

SD, Standard deviation; *CI-Up.*, 95% upper confidence limit; *CI-Lo.*, 95% lower confidence limit; *Med.*, median; *Max.*, maximum; *Min.*, minimum; *Lo.Q.*, lower quartile; *Up.Qt.*, upper quartile; *RR-Lo.L*, lower limit of reference range; *RR-Up.L*, upper limit of reference range.

Table 175. Clinical chemistry: fasting baseline, men aged 20–29 years, SI units (7:00–9:00 A.M.)

	n	Mean	SD	CI-Up.	CI-Lo.	Med.	Max.	Min.	Lo.Qt.	Up.Qt.	RR-Lo.L	RR-Up.L
Alkaline phosphatase (U/l)	1159	95.11	22.73	96.42	93.80	92	172	31	78	111	57	143
AST (SGOT; U/l)	1049	9.69	3.47	9.90	9.48	9	49	4	8	11	6	18
ALT (SGPT; U/l)	1048	10.27	5.08	10.58	9.96	9	61	3	7	12	5	22
γ-GT (U/l)	1048	10.26	5.06	10.57	9.96	9	79	2	7	12	5	25
LDH (U/l)	1068	156.04	46.02	158.80	153.28	147	411	15	129	173	93	265
Total bilirubin (µmol/l)	923	8.90	4.32	9.18	8.62	8.21	27.37	1.71	5.47	11.63	3.42	18.81
Creatinine (µmol/l)	1171	73.97	10.71	74.59	73.36	72.49	109.62	34.48	67.18	79.56	58.34	99.01
Blood urea (BUN; mmol/l)	951	4.85	1.30	4.93	4.77	4.83	9.66	1.67	4.00	5.66	2.50	7.66
Uric acid (µmol/l)	774	316.98	60.29	321.22	312.73	315.3	690.0	148.7	273.6	356.9	202.3	428.3
Total protein (g/l)	1164	72.45	5.51	72.77	72.14	71	93	50	70	76	60	83
Total cholesterol (mmol/l)	1141	4.76	0.89	4.81	4.71	4.7	10.8	2.5	4.2	5.3	3.15	6.55
Triglycerides (mmol/l)	888	1.31	0.68	1.36	1.27	1.13	5.14	0.27	0.83	1.64	0.50	3.15
Glucose fasting (mmol/l)	1146	5.05	0.59	5.08	5.01	5.00	7.71	3.01	4.72	5.38	3.89	6.33
Calcium (mmol/l)	611	2.34	0.13	2.35	2.33	2.36	2.60	1.82	2.28	2.43	2.04	2.56
Sodium (mmol/l)	1076	143.69	2.95	143.87	143.52	143.7	157.0	135.1	142.0	145.5	138.1	149.2
Potassium (mmol/l)	1161	4.36	0.34	4.38	4.34	4.35	5.98	3.44	4.10	4.59	3.72	5.10
Chloride (mmol/l)	1027	106.03	4.89	106.33	105.73	105.9	127.0	89.0	102.9	108.8	97.8	118.0
Age (years)	1171	25.72	2.42	–	–	–	29	20	–	–	–	–

SD, Standard deviation; CI-Up, 95% upper confidence limit; CI-Lo, 95% lower confidence limit; Med., median; Max., maximum; Min., minimum; Lo.Q., lower quartile; Up.Qt., upper quartile; RR-Lo.L, lower limit of reference range; RR-Up.L, upper limit of reference range.

Table 176. Clinical chemistry: fasting baseline, men aged 30–39 years, conventional units (7:00–9:00 A.M.)

	n	Mean	SD	CI-Up.	CI-Lo.	Med.	Max.	Min.	Lo.Qt.	Up.Qt.	RR-Lo.L	RR-Up.L
Alkaline phosphatase (U/l)	325	95.84	24.87	98.54	93.13	92	188	44	78	109	61	164
AST (SGOT; U/l)	285	9.02	2.58	9.32	8.72	9	25	5	8	10	6	15
ALT (SGPT; U/l)	285	10.18	5.21	10.78	9.57	9	53	3	7	12	5	21
γ-GT (U/l)	285	10.27	3.94	10.73	9.82	9	28	4	8	12	6	21
LDH (U/l)	278	147.15	28.92	150.55	143.75	143	299	93	128	160	106	215
Total bilirubin (mg/dl)	233	0.49	0.21	0.52	0.46	0.45	1.11	0.13	0.35	0.60	0.20	0.91
Creatinine (mg/dl)	328	0.82	0.11	0.83	0.81	0.82	1.19	0.40	0.76	0.87	0.64	1.09
Blood urea (BUN; mg/dl)	225	31.37	8.17	32.44	30.30	29	83	17	26	35	21	51
Uric acid (mg/dl)	290	5.36	0.92	5.46	5.25	5.3	7.7	3.1	4.7	6.0	3.8	7.3
Total protein (g/dl)	325	7.28	0.44	7.32	7.23	7.3	9.6	6.2	7.0	7.5	6.5	8.2
Total cholesterol (mg/dl)	308	201.79	28.26	204.94	198.63	201	292	111	182	220	152	262
Triglycerides (mg/dl)	217	110.03	46.05	116.15	103.90	103	278	36	76	133	45	229
Glucose fasting (mg/dl)	312	92.73	9.37	93.77	91.69	92	129	68	87	98	77	115
Calcium (mmol/l)	228	2.35	0.10	2.37	2.34	2.36	2.60	1.95	2.30	2.41	2.18	2.52
Sodium (mmol/l)	299	143.35	2.48	143.63	143.07	144.2	149.8	137.2	142.0	145.1	138.2	147.8
Potassium (mmol/l)	319	4.39	0.35	4.43	4.35	4.36	6.63	3.60	4.18	4.59	3.80	5.08
Chloride (mmol/l)	269	104.86	3.84	105.32	104.40	105.0	121.2	95.0	101.8	107.1	98.1	112.3
Age (years)	328	32.8	2.3	–	–	–	39	30	–	–	–	–

SD, Standard deviation; CI-Up., 95% upper confidence limit; CI-Lo., 95% lower confidence limit; Med., median; Max., maximum; Min., minimum; Lo.Q., lower quartile; Up.Qt., upper quartile; RR-Lo.L, lower limit of reference range; RR-Up.L, upper limit of reference range.

Table 177. Clinical chemistry: fasting baseline, men aged 30–39 years, SI units (7:00–9:00 A.M.)

	n	Mean	SD	CI-Up.	CI-Lo.	Med.	Max.	Min.	Lo.Qt.	Up.Qt.	RR-Lo.L	RR-Up.L
Alkaline phosphatase (U/l)	325	95.84	24.87	98.54	93.13	92.0	188.0	44.0	78.0	109.0	61.0	164.0
AST (SGOT; U/l)	285	9.02	2.58	9.32	8.72	9.0	25.0	5.0	8.0	10.0	6.0	15.0
ALT (SGPT; U/l)	285	10.18	5.21	10.78	9.57	9.0	53.0	3.0	7.0	12.0	5.0	21.0
γ-GT (U/l)	285	10.27	3.94	10.73	9.82	9.0	28.0	4.0	8.0	12.0	6.0	21.0
LDH (U/l)	278	147.15	28.92	150.55	143.75	143.0	299.0	93.0	128.0	160.0	106.0	215.0
Total bilirubin (μmol/l)	233	8.38	3.51	8.83	7.93	7.70	18.99	2.22	5.99	10.26	3.42	15.56
Creatinine (μmol/l)	328	72.71	9.89	73.78	71.64	72.49	105.20	35.36	67.18	76.91	56.58	96.36
Blood urea (BUN; mmol/l)	225	5.22	1.36	5.40	5.05	4.83	13.82	2.83	4.33	5.83	3.50	8.49
Uric acid (μmol/l)	290	318.63	54.71	324.93	312.34	315.3	458.0	184.4	279.6	356.9	226.0	434.2
Total protein (g/l)	325	72.75	4.44	73.24	72.27	73.0	96.0	62.0	70.0	75.0	65.0	82.0
Total cholesterol (mmol/l)	308	5.21	0.73	5.29	5.12	5.19	7.53	2.86	4.70	5.68	3.92	6.76
Triglycerides (mmol/l)	217	1.25	0.52	1.32	1.18	1.17	3.17	0.41	0.87	1.52	0.51	2.61
Glucose fasting (mmol/l)	312	5.15	0.52	5.20	5.09	5.11	7.16	3.77	4.83	5.44	4.27	6.38
Calcium (mmol/l)	228	2.35	0.10	2.37	2.34	2.36	2.60	1.95	2.30	2.41	2.18	2.52
Sodium (mmol/l)	299	143.35	2.48	143.63	143.07	143.60	149.90	137.00	142.00	145.10	138.20	147.80
Potassium (mmol/l)	319	4.39	0.35	4.43	4.35	4.36	6.63	3.60	4.18	4.59	3.80	5.08
Chloride (mmol/l)	269	104.86	3.84	105.32	104.40	104.80	121.00	94.80	102.40	107.10	98.10	112.30
Age (years)	328	32.8	2.3	–	–	–	39	30	–	–	–	–

SD, Standard deviation; *CI-Up.*, 95% upper confidence limit; *CI-Lo.*, 95% lower confidence limit; *Med.*, median; *Max.*, maximum; *Min.*, minimum; *Lo.Q.*, lower quartile; *Up.Qt.*, upper quartile; *RR-Lo.L*, lower limit of reference range; *RR-Up.L*, upper limit of reference range.

6.6.2 Changes After Repeated Measurements

6.6.2.1 Elderly Subjects

Table 178. Clinical chemistry: changes after 24 h, differences from baseline, men and women aged 50–80 years, conventional units

	n	Mean	SD	CI-Up.	CI-Lo.	Min.	Max.	Med.	RR-Lo.L	RR-Up.L	D_{crit}
Alkaline phosphatase (U/l)	105	-3.47	12.22	-1.13	-5.80	-43	26	-2	-41	20	23.99
AST (SGOT; U/l)	125	0.39	2.87	0.89	-0.11	-5	11	0	-5	9	5.57
ALT (SGPT; U/l)	125	-0.16	2.03	0.20	-0.52	-7	8	0	-4	6	3.98
γ-GT (U/l)	125	-0.24	1.39	0.00	-0.48	-5	3	0	-3	3	2.70
LDH (U/l)	79	1.01	19.72	5.36	-3.34	-45	41	3	-39	40	38.49
Total bilirubin (mg/dl)	125	-0.03	0.13	-0.01	-0.05	-0.29	0.25	-0.02	-0.27	0.22	0.23
Creatinine (mg/dl)	105	0.00	0.05	0.01	-0.01	-0.12	0.15	0.00	-0.11	0.11	0.10
Uric acid (mg/dl)	125	-0.01	0.48	0.07	-0.1	-1.1	1.1	0.	-0.9	1.0	0.91
Total cholesterol (mg/dl)	115	3.02	13.57	5.50	0.54	-34	31	2	-19	29	26.41
Triglycerides (mg/dl)	105	1.17	18.01	4.61	-2.28	-37	34	3	-34	33	31.61
Glucose fasting (mg/dl)	125	-0.15	13.70	2.25	-2.55	-98	46	0	-23	19	23.88
Sodium (mmol/l)	125	0.12	2.10	0.48	-0.25	-3.1	3.7	0.0	-3.1	3.7	4.02
Potassium (mmol/l)	125	0.20	0.50	0.28	0.11	-0.81	2.40	0.14	-0.66	0.86	0.81
Chloride (mmol/l)	109	0.83	2.84	1.36	0.29	-5.0	9.3	0.4	-3.8	9.3	5.41
Age (years)	125	67.0	5.8	–	–	50	77	–	–	–	–

SD, Standard deviation; *CI-Up.*, 95% upper confidence limit; *CI-Lo.*, 95% lower confidence limit; *Med*, median; *Max.*, maximum; *Min.*, minimum; *RR-Lo.L*, lower limit of reference range; *RR-Up.L*, upper limit of reference range; D_{crit} critical difference 0.05.

Table 179. Clinical chemistry: changes after 24 h, differences from baseline, men and women aged 50–80 years, SI units

	n	Mean	SD	CI-Up.	CI-Lo.	Min.	Max.	Med.	RR-Lo.L	RR-Up.L	D$_{crit}$
Alkaline phosphatase (U/l)	105	-3.47	12.22	-1.13	-5.80	-43	26	-2	-41	20	23.99
AST (SGOT; U/l)	125	0.39	2.87	0.89	-0.11	-5	11	0	-5	9	5.57
ALT (SGPT; U/l)	125	-0.16	2.03	0.20	-0.52	-7	8	0	-4	6	3.98
γ-GT (U/l)	125	-0.24	1.39	0.00	-0.48	-5	3	0	-3	3	2.70
LDH (U/l)	79	1.01	19.72	5.36	-3.34	-45	41	3	-39	40	38.49
Total bilirubin (µmol/l)	125	-0.54	2.17	-0.16	-0.92	-4.96	4.28	-0.34	-4.62	3.76	3.95
Creatinine (µmol/l)	105	-0.05	4.57	0.82	-0.92	-10.61	13.26	0.00	-9.72	9.72	8.81
Uric acid (µmol/l)	125	-0.67	28.67	4.36	-5.69	-65.43	65.43	0.00	-53.54	59.49	54.06
Total cholesterol (mmol/l)	115	0.08	0.35	0.14	0.01	-0.88	0.80	0.05	-0.49	0.75	0.68
Triglycerides (mmol/l)	105	0.01	0.21	0.05	-0.03	-0.42	0.39	0.03	-0.39	0.38	0.36
Glucose fasting (mmol/l)	125	-0.01	0.76	0.12	-0.14	-5.44	2.55	0.00	-1.28	1.05	1.33
Sodium (mmol/l)	125	0.12	2.10	0.48	-0.25	-3.1	3.7	0.0	-3.1	3.7	4.02
Potassium (mmol/l)	125	0.20	0.50	0.28	0.11	-0.81	2.40	0.14	-0.66	0.86	0.81
Chloride (mmol/l)	109	0.83	2.84	1.36	0.29	-5.0	9.3	0.	-3.8	9.3	5.41
Age (years)	125	67.0	5.8	–	–	50	77	–	–	–	–

SD, Standard deviation; *CI-Up.*, 95% upper confidence limit; *CI-Lo.*, 95% lower confidence limit; *Med.*, median; *Max.*, maximum; *Min.*, minimum; *RR-Lo.L*, lower limit of reference range; *RR-Up.L*, upper limit of reference range; *D$_{crit}$*, critical difference 0.05.

Table 180. Clinical chemistry: changes after 48 h, differences from baseline, men and women aged 50–80 years, conventional units

	n	Mean	SD	CI-Up.	CI-Lo.	Min.	Max.	Med.	RR-Lo.L	RR-Up.L	D_{crit}
Alkaline phosphatase (U/l)	127	0.69	6.49	1.82	-0.44	-12	16	1	-12	13	12.67
AST (SGOT; U/l)	131	-0.42	2.41	-0.01	-0.83	-6	9	0	-5	4	4.44
ALT (SGPT; U/l)	141	0.07	1.70	0.35	-0.21	-4	8	0	-3	3	3.26
γ-GT (U/l)	141	-0.11	1.39	0.12	-0.34	-4	3	0	-3	2	2.72
LDH (U/l)	123	-4.58	20.91	-0.88	-8.27	-60	68	-2	-52	31	40.01
Total bilirubin (mg/dl)	141	-0.02	0.14	0.00	-0.05	-0.52	0.29	-0.02	-0.33	0.25	0.25
Creatinine (mg/dl)	113	-0.01	0.05	0.00	-0.02	-0.13	0.14	-0.01	-0.1	0.09	0.09
Uric acid (mg/dl)	141	-0.05	0.56	0.04	-0.15	-2.1	2	0	-1.2	0.9	1.11
Total cholesterol (mg/dl)	141	-1.10	13.49	1.13	-3.33	-35	35	-1	-29	25	26.11
Triglycerides (mg/dl)	141	-0.64	18.04	2.69	-3.96	-54	46	-2	-44	27	32.78
Glucose fasting (mg/dl)	141	-1.33	7.82	-0.04	-2.62	-23	17	-1	-16	12	14.82
Sodium (mmol/l)	141	0.20	2.22	0.57	-0.16	-6.2	5.5	0.2	-4.3	4.5	4.28
Potassium (mmol/l)	141	0.02	0.39	0.08	-0.05	-1.08	1.34	-0.01	-0.8	0.89	0.77
Chloride (mmol/l)	123	0.90	2.68	1.35	0.46	-4	11.4	0.6	-3.1	6.3	4.78
Age (years)	141	65.6	5.9	–	–	50	77	–	–	–	–

SD, Standard deviation; CI-Up., 95% upper confidence limit; CI-Lo., 95% lower confidence limit; Med., median; Max., maximum; Min., minimum; RR-Lo.L, lower limit of reference range; RR-Up.L, upper limit of reference range; D_{crit}, critical difference 0.05.

Table 181. Clinical chemistry: changes after 48 h, differences from baseline, men and women aged 50–80 years, SI units

	n	Mean	SD	CI-Up.	CI-Lo.	Min.	Max.	Med.	RR-Lo.L	RR-Up.L	D_{crit}
Alkaline phosphatase (U/l)	127	0.69	6.49	1.82	-0.44	-12	16	1	-12	13	12.67
AST (SGOT; U/l)	131	-0.42	2.41	-0.01	-0.83	-6	9	0	-5	4	4.44
ALT (SGPT; U/l)	141	0.07	1.70	0.35	-0.21	-4	8	0	-3	3	3.26
γ-GT (U/l)	141	-0.11	1.39	0.12	-0.34	-4	3	0	-3	2	2.72
LDH (U/l)	123	-4.58	20.91	-0.88	-8.27	-60	68	-2	-52	31	40.01
Total bilirubin (µmol/l)	141	-0.40	2.48	0.01	-0.81	-8.89	4.96	-0.34	-5.64	4.28	4.29
Creatinine (µmol/l)	113	-1.02	4.23	-0.25	-1.80	-11.49	12.38	-0.88	-8.84	7.96	8.14
Uric acid (µmol/l)	141	-3.12	33.56	2.42	-8.66	-124.92	118.97	0.00	-71.38	53.54	65.91
Total cholesterol (mmol/l)	141	-0.03	0.35	0.03	-0.09	-0.90	0.90	-0.03	-0.75	0.65	0.67
Triglycerides (mmol/l)	141	-0.01	0.21	0.03	-0.04	-0.62	0.52	-0.02	-0.50	0.31	0.37
Glucose fasting (mmol/l)	141	-0.07	0.43	0.00	-0.15	-1.28	0.94	-0.06	-0.89	0.67	0.82
Sodium (mmol/l)	141	0.20	2.22	0.57	-0.16	-6.2	5.5	0.2	-4.3	4.5	4.28
Potassium (mmol/l)	141	0.02	0.39	0.08	-0.05	-1.08	1.34	-0.01	-0.80	0.89	0.77
Chloride (mmol/l)	123	0.90	2.68	1.35	0.46	-4.0	11.4	0.6	-3.1	6.3	4.78
Age (years)	141	65.6	5.9	–	–	50	77	–	–	–	–

SD, Standard deviation; *CI-Up.*, 95% upper confidence limit; *CI-Lo.*, 95% lower confidence limit; *Med.*, median; *Max.*, maximum; *Min.*, minimum; *RR-Lo.L*, lower limit of reference range; *RR-Up.L*, upper limit of reference range; D_{crit} critical difference 0.05.

Table 182. Clinical chemistry: changes after 1 week, differences from baseline, men and women aged 50–80 years, conventional units

	n	Mean	SD	CI-Up.	CI-Lo.	Min.	Max.	Med.	RR-Lo.L	RR-Up.L	D_{crit}
Alkaline phosphatase (U/l)	262	1.47	8.16	2.46	0.48	-18	21	2	-15	16	15.30
AST (SGOT; U/l)	263	-0.22	2.25	0.06	-0.49	-9	11	0	-5	4	4.70
ALT (SGPT; U/l)	259	-0.06	2.08	0.19	-0.31	-9	9	0	-5	3	3.63
γ-GT (U/l)	263	-0.07	1.84	0.15	-0.29	-8	9	0	-4	4	4.14
LDH (U/l)	213	-2.69	23.40	0.45	-5.83	-81	75	-2	-61	46	48.70
Total bilirubin (mg/dl)	263	0.00	0.15	0.01	-0.02	-0.38	0.61	0	-0.3	0.28	0.27
Creatinine (mg/dl)	263	0.01	0.08	0.01	0.00	-0.23	0.25	0	-0.15	0.16	0.15
Uric acid (mg/dl)	263	0.10	0.63	0.17	0.02	-1.9	2.3	0.1	-1.1	1.4	1.32
Total cholesterol (mg/dl)	233	0.78	16.90	2.95	-1.39	-45	65	-1	-29	34	32.70
Triglycerides (mg/dl)	233	0.12	11.52	1.60	-1.36	-39	36	1	-20	23	20.30
Glucose fasting (mg/dl)	256	0.79	8.86	1.88	-0.29	-28	34	0	-17	18	16.30
Sodium (mmol/l)	263	0.01	1.00	0.13	-0.11	-2.9	3	0	-1.8	1.7	1.65
Potassium (mmol/l)	263	-0.01	0.28	0.03	-0.04	-0.74	0.91	0	-0.6	0.59	0.49
Chloride (mmol/l)	263	0.33	2.26	0.61	0.06	-5.5	5.6	0.5	-3.9	4.1	3.01
Age (years)	263	67.5	5.8	–	–	50	80	–	–	–	–

SD, Standard deviation; *CI-Up.*, 95% upper confidence limit; *CI-Lo.*, 95% lower confidence limit; *Med.*, median; *Max.*, maximum; *Min.*, minimum; *RR-Lo.L*, lower limit of reference range; *RR-Up.L*, upper limit of reference range; D_{crit} critical difference 0.05.

Table 183. Clinical chemistry: changes after 1 week, differences from baseline, men and women aged 50–80 years, SI units

	n	Mean	SD	CI-Up.	CI-Lo.	Min.	Max.	Med.	RR-Lo.L	RR-Up.L	D_crit
Alkaline phosphatase (U/l)	262	1.47	8.16	2.46	0.48	-18	21	2	-15	16	15.30
AST (SGOT; U/l)	263	-0.22	2.25	0.06	-0.49	-9	11	0	-5	4	4.70
ALT (SGPT; U/l)	259	-0.06	2.08	0.19	-0.31	-9	9	0	-5	3	3.63
γ-GT (U/l)	263	-0.07	1.84	0.15	-0.29	-8	9	0	-4	4	4.14
LDH (U/l)	213	-2.69	23.40	0.45	-5.83	-81.0	75.0	-2.0	-61.0	46.0	48.70
Total bilirubin (μmol/l)	263	-0.06	2.51	0.25	-0.36	-6.50	10.43	0.00	-5.13	4.79	4.58
Creatinine (μmol/l)	263	0.49	6.85	1.32	-0.34	-20.33	22.10	0.00	-13.26	14.14	13.26
Uric acid (μmol/l)	263	5.77	37.36	10.28	1.25	-113.02	136.82	5.95	-65.43	83.28	78.52
Total cholesterol (mmol/l)	233	0.02	0.44	0.08	-0.04	-1.16	1.68	-0.03	-0.75	0.88	0.84
Triglycerides (mmol/l)	233	0.00	0.13	0.02	-0.02	-0.44	0.41	0.01	-0.23	0.26	0.23
Glucose fasting (mmol/l)	256	0.04	0.49	0.10	-0.02	-1.55	1.89	0.00	-0.94	1.00	0.90
Sodium (mmol/l)	263	0.01	1.00	0.13	-0.11	-2.9	3.0	0.0	-1.8	1.7	1.65
Potassium (mmol/l)	263	-0.01	0.28	0.03	-0.04	-0.74	0.91	0.00	-0.60	0.59	0.49
Chloride (mmol/l)	263	0.33	2.26	0.61	0.06	-5.5	5.6	0.5	-3.9	4.1	3.01
Age (years)	263	67.5	5.8	–	–	50	80	–	–	–	–

SD, Standard deviation; *CI-Up*, 95% upper confidence limit; *CI-Lo*, 95% lower confidence limit; *Med.*, median; *Max.*, maximum; *Min.*, minimum; *RR-Lo.L*, lower limit of reference range; *RR-Up.L*, upper limit of reference range; *D_crit*, critical difference 0.05.

Table 184. Clinical chemistry: changes after 2 weeks, differences from baseline, men and women aged 50–80 years, conventional units

	n	Mean	SD	CI-Up.	CI-Lo.	Min.	Max.	Med.	RR-Lo.L	RR-Up.L	D_{crit}
Alkaline phosphatase (U/l)	193	1.68	11.28	3.27	0.09	−34	30	2	−23	21	21.92
AST (SGOT; U/l)	215	−0.18	2.84	0.20	−0.56	−10	15	0	−8	5	5.27
ALT (SGPT; U/l)	215	−0.37	2.85	0.01	−0.75	−14	11	0	−9	4	5.51
γ-GT (U/l)	195	−0.15	2.86	0.25	−0.55	−15	14	0	−6	5	5.59
LDH (U/l)	171	−1.33	36.98	4.21	−6.88	−94	96	0	−86	77	67.61
Total bilirubin (mg/dl)	215	0.00	0.17	0.02	−0.03	−0.52	0.60	−0.02	−0.34	0.35	0.32
Creatinine (mg/dl)	215	0.01	0.09	0.02	−0.01	−0.31	0.36	0.00	−0.18	0.19	0.16
Uric acid (mg/dl)	215	0.14	0.64	0.23	0.05	−2.1	2.8	0.1	−1.1	1.5	1.21
Total cholesterol (mg/dl)	205	0.46	20.11	3.22	−2.29	−49	49	1	−37	36	38.73
Triglycerides (mg/dl)	184	2.71	17.80	5.28	0.13	−38	50	−0.5	−29	35	32.62
Glucose fasting (mg/dl)	214	0.35	10.80	1.80	−1.10	−27	49	0	−20	23	18.91
Sodium (mmol/l)	203	0.14	1.81	0.39	−0.11	−6.9	6.7	0.0	−3.2	2.8	3.43
Potassium (mmol/l)	215	0.09	0.44	0.15	0.04	−1.76	1.17	0.07	−0.94	0.91	0.83
Chloride (mmol/l)	195	0.25	3.01	0.67	−0.17	−6.7	6.8	0.2	−5.8	5.8	5.37
Age (years)	215	66.2	5.8	–	–	50	80	–	–	–	–

SD, Standard deviation; *CI-Up*, 95% upper confidence limit; *CI-Lo*, 95% lower confidence limit; *Med.*, median; *Max.*, maximum; *Min.*, minimum; *RR-Lo.L*, lower limit of reference range; *RR-Up.L*, upper limit of reference range; D_{crit}, critical difference 0.05.

Table 185. Clinical chemistry: changes after 2 weeks, differences from baseline, men and women aged 50–80 years, SI units

	n	Mean	SD	CI-Up.	CI-Lo.	Min.	Max.	Med.	RR-Lo.L	RR-Up.L	D_crit
Alkaline phosphatase (U/l)	193	1.68	11.28	3.27	0.09	−34	30	2	−23	21	21.92
AST (SGOT; U/l)	215	−0.18	2.84	0.20	−0.56	−10	15	0	−8	5	5.27
ALT (SGPT; U/l)	215	−0.37	2.85	0.01	−0.75	−14	11	0	−9	4	5.51
γ-GT (U/l)	195	−0.15	2.86	0.25	−0.55	−15	14	0	−6	5	5.59
LDH (U/l)	171	−1.33	36.98	4.21	−6.88	−94.0	96.0	0.0	−86.0	77.0	67.61
Total bilirubin (µmol/l)	215	−0.05	2.94	0.34	−0.45	−8.89	10.26	−0.34	−5.82	5.99	5.44
Creatinine (µmol/l)	215	0.50	7.56	1.51	−0.51	−27.40	31.82	0.00	−15.91	16.80	14.11
Uric acid (µmol/l)	215	8.33	38.31	13.45	3.21	−124.92	166.56	5.95	−65.43	89.23	71.86
Total cholesterol (mmol/l)	205	0.01	0.52	0.08	−0.06	−1.26	1.26	0.03	−0.95	0.93	1.00
Triglycerides (mmol/l)	184	0.03	0.20	0.06	0.00	−0.43	0.57	−0.01	−0.33	0.40	0.37
Glucose fasting (mmol/l)	214	0.02	0.60	0.10	−0.06	−1.50	2.72	0.00	−1.11	1.28	1.05
Sodium (mmol/l)	203	0.14	1.81	0.39	−0.11	−6.9	6.7	0.0	−3.2	2.8	3.43
Potassium (mmol/l)	215	0.09	0.44	0.15	0.04	−1.76	1.17	0.07	−0.94	0.91	0.83
Chloride (mmol/l)	195	0.25	3.01	0.67	−0.17	−6.7	6.8	0.2	−5.8	5.8	5.37
Age (years)	215	66.2	5.8	–	–	50	80	–	–	–	–

SD, Standard deviation; *CI-Up.*, 95% upper confidence limit; *CI-Lo.*, 95% lower confidence limit; *Med.*, median; *Max.*, maximum; *Min.*, minimum; *RR-Lo.L*, lower limit of reference range; *RR-Up.L*, upper limit of reference range; *D_crit* critical difference 0.05.

6.6.2.2 Young Subjects

Table 186. Clinical chemistry: changes after 24 h, differences from baseline, men and women aged 20–39 years, conventional units

	n	Mean	SD	CI-Up.	CI-Lo.	Min.	Max.	Med.	RR-Lo.L	RR-Up.L	D_{crit}
Alkaline phosphatase (U/l)	281	0.91	13.69	2.51	-0.69	-71	95	1	-25	23	21.85
AST (SGOT; U/l)	261	0.27	2.69	0.60	-0.05	-14	13	0	-4	6	4.34
ALT (SGPT; U/l)	261	0.62	3.27	1.01	0.22	-8	23	0	-5	7	5.32
γ-GT (U/l)	261	0.82	1.66	1.02	0.61	-8	10	1	-1	5	3.34
LDH (U/l)	257	-1.98	38.09	2.68	-6.63	-136	113	1	-93	87	56.89
Total bilirubin (mg/dl)	254	0.01	0.38	0.06	-0.03	-1.11	1.52	-0.01	-0.68	0.70	0.66
Creatinine (mg/dl)	284	0.01	0.13	0.02	-0.01	-0.38	0.36	0.00	-0.26	0.30	0.24
Uric acid (mg/dl)	189	-0.14	0.77	-0.03	-0.25	-2.00	2.00	-0.10	-1.70	1.40	1.52
Total cholesterol (mg/dl)	279	2.47	18.39	4.63	0.31	-42	48	3	-34	38	33.89
Glucose fasting (mg/dl)	282	-0.99	11.55	0.36	-2.34	-30	31	-1	-24	25	19.22
Sodium (mmol/l)	281	0.02	1.39	0.19	-0.14	-1.93	1.99	0.01	-2.71	1.84	1.89
Potassium (mmol/l)	203	-0.03	0.39	0.03	-0.08	-0.91	0.94	-0.01	-0.71	0.89	0.73
Age (years)	284	27.5	3.6	–	–	21	39	–	–	–	–

SD, Standard deviation; CI-Up., 95% upper confidence limit; CI-Lo., 95% lower confidence limit; Med., median; Max., maximum; Min., minimum; RR-Lo.L, lower limit of reference range; RR-Up.L, upper limit of reference range; D_{crit}, critical difference 0.05.

Table 187. Clinical chemistry: changes after 24 h, differences from baseline, men and women aged 20–39 years, SI units

	n	Mean	SD	CI-Up.	CI-Lo.	Min.	Max.	Med.	RR-Lo.L	RR-Up.L	D_{crit}
Alkaline phosphatase (U/l)	281	0.91	13.69	2.51	-0.69	-71	95	1	-25	23	21.85
AST (SGOT; U/l)	261	0.27	2.69	0.60	-0.05	-14	13	0	-4	6	4.34
ALT (SGPT; U/l)	261	0.62	3.27	1.01	0.22	-8	23	0	-5	7	5.32
γ-GT (U/l)	261	0.82	1.66	1.02	0.61	-8	10	1	-1	5	3.34
LDH (U/l)	257	-1.98	38.09	2.68	-6.63	-136.00	113.00	1.00	-93.00	87.00	56.89
Total bilirubin (µmol/l)	254	0.24	6.43	1.03	-0.56	-19.02	26.05	-0.25	-11.60	11.92	11.35
Creatinine (µmol/l)	284	0.45	11.69	1.81	-0.91	-33.59	31.82	0.00	-22.98	26.52	21.00
Uric acid (µmol/l)	189	-8.09	45.59	-1.59	-14.59	-118.97	118.97	-5.95	-101.12	83.28	90.31
Total cholesterol (mmol/l)	279	0.06	0.47	0.12	0.01	-1.08	1.24	0.08	-0.88	0.98	0.87
Glucose fasting (mg/dl)	282	-0.06	0.64	0.02	-0.13	-1.67	1.72	-0.06	-1.33	1.39	1.07
Sodium (mmol/l)	281	0.02	1.39	0.19	-0.14	-1.93	1.99	0.01	-2.71	1.84	1.89
Potassium (mmol/l)	203	-0.03	0.39	0.03	-0.08	-0.91	0.94	-0.01	-0.71	0.89	0.73
Age (years)	284	27.5	3.6	–	–	21	39	–	–	–	–

SD, Standard deviation; *CI-Up.*, 95% upper confidence limit; *CI-Lo.*, 95% lower confidence limit; *Med.*, median; *Max.*, maximum; *Min.*, minimum; *RR-Lo.L*, lower limit of reference range; *RR-Up.L*, upper limit of reference range; D_{crit}, critical difference 0.05.

Table 188. Clinical chemistry: changes after 1 week, differences from baseline, men and women aged 20–39 years, conventional units

	n	Mean	SD	CI-Up.	CI-Lo.	Min.	Max.	Med.	RR-Lo.L	RR-Up.L	D_{crit}
Alkaline phosphatase (U/l)	203	0.59	6.87	1.53	-0.36	0	26	-25	-12	17	13.16
AST (SGOT; U/l)	203	0.00	1.56	0.21	-0.21	0	9	-4	-2	3	3.04
ALT (SGPT; U/l)	203	0.29	1.95	0.55	0.02	0	9	-4	-3	5	3.57
γ-GT (U/l)	203	-0.89	1.27	-0.71	-1.06	-1	3	-7	-4	2	2.37
LDH (U/l)	199	0.46	17.29	2.86	-1.95	2	54	-75	-46	39	33.24
Total bilirubin (mg/dl)	202	0.01	0.34	0.06	-0.03	-0.01	0.15	-0.10	-0.08	0.13	0.12
Creatinine (mg/dl)	203	0.00	0.07	0.01	-0.01	0.00	0.20	-0.26	-0.14	0.17	0.13
Uric acid (mg/dl)	145	0.03	0.63	0.13	-0.07	0.00	1.50	-2.00	-1.00	1.20	1.23
Total cholesterol (mg/dl)	203	-0.15	10.14	1.25	-1.54	1	29	-28	-22	20	19.73
Glucose fasting (mg/dl)	203	0.79	5.80	1.59	-0.01	1	16	-16	-10	12	10.95
Sodium (mmol/l)	203	0.00	0.71	0.10	-0.10	0.00	1.89	-2.40	-1.10	1.41	1.24
Potassium (mmol/l)	203	-0.02	0.33	0.03	-0.06	-0.01	0.92	-0.80	-0.65	0.61	0.64
Age (years)	203	27.4	3.4	–	–	–	37	21	–	–	–

SD, Standard deviation; *CI-Up.*, 95% upper confidence limit; *CI-Lo.*, 95% lower confidence limit; *Med.*, median; *Max.*, maximum; *Min.*, minimum; *RR-Lo.L*, lower limit of reference range; *RR-Up.L*, upper limit of reference range; D_{crit}, critical difference 0.05.

Table 189. Clinical chemistry: changes after 1 week, differences from baseline, men and women aged 20–39 years, SI units

	n	Mean	SD	CI-Up.	CI-Lo.	Min.	Max.	Med.	RR-Lo.L	RR-Up.L	D_{crit}
Alkaline phosphatase (U/l)	203	0.59	6.87	1.53	-0.36	0	26	-25	-12	17	13.16
AST (SGOT; U/l)	203	0.00	1.56	0.21	-0.21	0	9	-4	-2	3	3.04
ALT (SGPT; U/l)	203	0.29	1.95	0.55	0.02	0	9	-4	-3	5	3.57
γ-GT (U/l)	203	-0.89	1.27	-0.71	-1.06	-1	3	-7	-4	2	2.37
LDH (U/l)	199	0.46	17.29	2.86	-1.95	2	54	-75	-46	39	33.24
Total bilirubin (μmol/l)	202	0.26	5.75	1.05	-0.54	-0.25	2.52	-1.73	-1.37	2.22	2.05
Creatinine (μmol/l)	203	-0.05	6.03	0.78	-0.88	0.00	17.68	-22.98	-12.38	15.03	11.85
Uric acid (μmol/l)	145	1.81	37.45	7.90	-4.29	0.00	89.23	-118.97	-59.49	71.38	73.11
Total cholesterol (mmol/l)	203	0.00	0.26	0.03	-0.04	0.03	0.75	-0.72	-0.57	0.52	0.51
Glucose fasting (mmol/l)	203	0.04	0.32	0.09	0.00	0.06	0.89	-0.89	-0.56	0.67	0.61
Sodium (mmol/l)	203	0.00	0.71	0.10	-0.10	0.00	1.89	-2.40	-1.10	1.41	1.24
Potassium (mmol/l)	203	-0.02	0.33	0.03	-0.06	-0.01	0.92	-0.80	-0.65	0.61	0.64
Age (years)	203	27.4	3.4	–	–	–	37	21	–	–	–

SD, Standard deviation; *CI-Up.*, 95% upper confidence limit; *CI-Lo.*, 95% lower confidence limit; *Med.*, median; *Max.*, maximum; *Min.*, minimum; *RR-Lo.L*, lower limit of reference range; *RR-Up.L*, upper limit of reference range; D_{crit}, critical difference 0.05.

6.7 Hematology

6.7.1 Baseline Values

6.7.1.1 Elderly Subjects

Table 190. Hematology: fasting baseline, men and women aged 50–80 years (7:00–9:00 A.M.)

	n	Mean	SD	CI-Up.	CI-Lo.	Med.	Max.	Min.	Lo.Qt.	Up.Qt.	RR-Lo.L	RR-Up.L
Leukocytes (10^9/l)	1102	6.49	1.45	6.58	6.41	6.1	13.9	4.4	5.5	7.1	4.8	10.4
Erythrocytes (10^{12}/l)	1102	4.60	0.37	4.63	4.58	4.61	5.74	3.65	4.32	4.88	3.94	5.32
Hemoglobin (g/dl)	1102	13.91	1.30	13.99	13.83	13.9	17.6	9.9	13.0	14.9	11.4	16.3
Hematocrit (%)	969	41.86	3.62	42.08	41.63	41.8	52.1	31.7	39.3	44.5	34.4	49.0
MCV (fl)	970	90.24	4.32	90.51	89.97	90.4	109.9	71.1	87.6	93.0	81.6	97.7
MCH (pg/cell)	902	30.25	1.68	30.36	30.14	30.3	37.8	22.0	29.4	31.3	26.0	33.1
MCHC (g Hb/dl Er.)	970	33.60	1.14	33.68	33.53	33.7	37.9	30.8	32.8	34.4	31.5	35.8
Platelets (thrombocytes; 10^9/l)	1100	248.19	60.15	251.75	244.64	239	524	142	206	282	156	405
Lymphocytes (%)	1090	33.58	7.81	34.04	33.11	33	59	10	28	39	20	49
Monocytes (%)	1102	3.44	2.37	3.58	3.30	3	11	0	2	5	0	9
Eosinophils (%)	1102	2.69	1.82	2.80	2.58	2	13	0	1	4	0	7
Basophils (%)	1102	0.53	0.64	0.56	0.49	0	4	0	0	1	0	2
Segmented neutrophils (%)	1089	59.60	8.13	60.08	59.11	60	85	33	54	65	44	75
Bands (%)	783	0.07	0.29	0.09	0.05	0	3	0	0	0	0	1
Reticulocytes (‰)	466	14.59	5.74	15.11	14.07	14	34	0	11	18	6	28
Quick's test (%)	953	113.54	11.75	114.29	112.79	113	152	82	106	121	93	138
Age (years)	1102	66.3	6.2	–	–	–	80	53	–	–	–	–

SD, Standard deviation; *CI-Up.*, 95% upper confidence limit; *CI-Lo.*, 95% lower confidence limit; *Med.*, median; *Max.*, maximum; *Min.*, minimum; *Lo.Q.*, lower quartile; *Up.Qt.*, upper quarter; *RR-Lo.L*, lower limit of reference range; *RR-Up.L*, upper limit of reference range; *MCV*, mean corpuscular volume; *MCH*, mean corpuscular hemoglobin; *MCHC*, mean corpuscular hemoglobin concentration.

Table 191. Hematology: fasting baseline, men aged 50–80 years (7:00–9:00 A.M.)

	n	Mean	SD	CI-Up.	CI-Lo.	Med.	Max.	Min.	Lo.Qt.	Up.Qt.	RR-Lo.L	RR-Up.L
Leukocytes (10⁹/l)	489	6.68	1.61	6.82	6.54	6.1	13.9	4.4	5.5	7.5	4.9	10.9
Erythrocytes (10¹²/l)	489	4.81	0.30	4.84	4.79	4.8	5.7	3.8	4.62	5.00	4.19	5.40
Hemoglobin (g/dl)	489	14.80	0.99	14.89	14.72	14.8	17.6	10.8	13.0	15.1	13.2	13.5
Hematocrit (%)	489	43.82	3.01	44.08	43.55	44.1	51.6	33.5	41.7	45.8	38.6	49.4
MCV (fl)	489	91.06	3.88	91.40	90.72	90.9	102.8	76.7	88.4	93.8	83.5	97.8
MCH (pg/cell)	457	30.78	1.40	30.90	30.65	30.8	34.7	25.4	29.9	31.7	28.0	33.3
MCHC (g Hb/dl Er.)	489	33.84	1.14	33.94	33.74	34.0	37.9	30.9	33.1	34.5	31.6	36.2
Platelets (thrombocytes; 10⁹/l)	487	233.34	53.16	238.07	228.62	228	451.0	142.0	195	265	152	364
Lymphocytes (%)	483	32.33	7.63	33.01	31.65	32	56	10	27	37	19	49
Monocytes (%)	489	4.05	2.64	4.28	3.82	4	11	0	2	6	0	10
Eosinophils (%)	489	2.98	1.93	3.15	2.81	3	11	0	2	4	0	8
Basophils (%)	489	0.54	0.65	0.60	0.48	0	4	0	0	1	0	2
Segmented neutrophils (%)	483	59.90	7.87	60.60	59.19	60	80	33	55	65	45	75
Bands (%)	396	0.08	0.33	0.12	0.05	0	3	0	0	0	0	1
Reticulocytes (‰)	244	15.28	6.08	16.04	14.52	14	34	0	11	19	6	29
Quick's test (%)	480	112.80	12.06	113.88	111.72	112	152	82	105	120	90	138
Age (years)	489	66.4	6.2	–	–	–	80	53	–	–	–	–

SD, Standard deviation; CI-Up., 95% upper confidence limit; CI-Lo, 95% lower confidence limit; Med, median; Max, maximum; Min, minimum; Lo.Q, lower quartile; Up.Qt, upper quarter; RR-Lo.L, lower limit of reference range; RR-Up.L, upper limit of reference range; MCV, mean corpuscular volume; MCH, mean corpuscular hemoglobin; MCHC, mean corpuscular hemoglobin concentration.

Table 192. Hematology: fasting baseline, women aged 50–80 years (7:00–9:00 A.M.)

	n	Mean	SD	CI-Up.	CI-Lo.	Med.	Max.	Min.	Lo.Qt.	Up.Qt.	RR-Lo.L	RR-Up.L
Leukocytes (10^9/l)	613	6.35	1.30	6.45	6.24	6.0	11.8	4.4	5.5	6.8	4.8	10.1
Erythrocytes (10^{12}/l)	613	4.44	0.33	4.46	4.41	4.4	5.74	3.65	4.21	4.64	3.89	5.14
Hemoglobin (g/dl)	613	13.20	1.04	13.28	13.11	13.2	16.5	9.9	12.5	13.9	11.2	15.4
Hematocrit (%)	480	39.86	3.04	40.13	39.59	39.7	52.1	31.7	37.8	41.9	34.0	45.9
MCV (fl)	481	89.41	4.59	89.82	89.00	89.7	109.9	71.1	86.9	92.2	80.0	97.7
MCH (pg/cell)	445	29.71	1.78	29.87	29.54	29.9	37.8	22.0	28.9	30.8	25.6	32.4
MCHC (g Hb/dl Er.)	481	33.37	1.10	33.46	33.27	33.4	36.1	30.8	32.5	34.2	31.3	35.4
Platelets (thrombocytes; 10^9/l)	613	259.99	62.76	264.96	255.02	246	524	151	216	295	173	418
Lymphocytes (%)	607	34.57	7.82	35.19	33.94	34	59	15	29	40	21	50
Monocytes (%)	613	2.95	2.00	3.11	2.79	3	9	0	1	4	0	7
Eosinophils (%)	613	2.46	1.69	2.59	2.32	2	13	0	1	3	0	6
Basophils (%)	613	0.52	0.63	0.57	0.47	0	3	0	0	1	0	2
Segmented neutrophils (%)	606	59.36	8.34	60.02	58.69	60	85	37	53	65	44	75
Bands (%)	387	0.05	0.25	0.07	0.02	0	3	0	0	0	0	1
Reticulocytes (‰)	222	13.82	5.24	14.51	13.14	13	31	4	10	17	6	26
Quick's test (%)	473	114.29	11.39	115.32	113.26	113	150	85	106	121	94	138
Age (years)	613	66.1	6.2	–	–	–	80	53	–	–	–	–

SD, Standard deviation; *CI-Up.*, 95% upper confidence limit; *CI-Lo*, 95% lower confidence limit; *Med.*, median; *Max.*, maximum; *Min.*, minimum; *Lo.Q*, lower quartile; *Up.Qt*, upper quarter; *RR-Lo.L*, lower limit of reference range; *RR-Up.L*, upper limit of reference range; *MCV*, mean corpuscular volume; *MCH*, mean corpuscular hemoglobin; *MCHC*, mean corpuscular hemoglobin concentration.

Table 193. Hematology: fasting baseline, men and women aged 50–59 years (7:00–9:00 A.M.)

	n	Mean	SD	CI-Up.	CI-Lo.	Med.	Max.	Min.	Lo.Qt.	Up.Qt.	RR-Lo.L	RR-Up.L
Leukocytes 10^9/l	322	6.53	1.60	6.70	6.36	6.1	13.9	4.4	5.4	7.4	4.7	10.9
Erythrocytes (10^{12}/l)	322	4.58	0.33	4.61	4.54	4.60	5.36	3.72	4.35	4.83	3.92	5.22
Hemoglobin (g/dl)	322	13.79	1.16	13.92	13.67	13.7	16.5	9.9	12.9	14.7	11.70	16.0
Hematocrit (%)	249	41.68	2.99	42.05	41.31	41.4	49.2	34.3	39.5	43.9	36.6	47.6
MCV (fl)	249	89.68	3.62	90.13	89.23	89.7	100.7	78.7	87.5	92.0	82.4	96.6
MCH (pg/cell)	248	30.23	1.30	30.40	30.07	30.3	34.7	25.8	29.5	31.0	27.0	33.3
MCHC (g Hb/dl Er.)	249	33.75	1.13	33.89	33.61	33.8	37.9	31.0	32.9	34.5	31.7	35.9
Platelets (thrombocytes; 10^9/l)	322	239.95	46.70	245.05	234.85	240	430	147	207	272	161	341
Lymphocytes (%)	316	34.46	7.73	35.31	33.61	34	59	16	30	39	21	49
Monocytes (%)	322	2.75	1.96	2.97	2.54	3	10	0	1	4	0	7
Eosinophils (%)	322	2.53	1.62	2.71	2.36	2	9	0	1	4	0	6
Basophils (%)	322	0.49	0.59	0.56	0.43	0	2	0	0	1	0	2
Segmented neutrophils (%)	316	59.59	8.27	60.50	58.68	59	79	39	54	65	45	76
Bands (%)	194	0.07	0.25	0.10	0.03	0	1	0	0	0	0	1
Reticulocytes (‰)	189	15.40	6.07	16.26	14.53	14	34	0	11	20	6	29
Quick's test (%)	246	114.78	11.40	116.20	113.35	114	150	87	108	122	95	146
Age (years)	322	56.9	1.5	–	–	–	59	53	–	–	–	–

SD, Standard deviation; *CI-Up.*, 95% upper confidence limit; *CI-Lo.*, 95% lower confidence limit; *Med.*, median; *Max.*, maximum; *Min.*, minimum; *Lo.Q.*, lower quartile; *Up.Qt.*, upper quarter; *RR-Lo.L*, lower limit of reference range; *RR-Up.L*, upper limit of reference range; *MCV*, mean corpuscular volume; *MCH*, mean corpuscular hemoglobin; *MCHC*, mean corpuscular hemoglobin concentration.

Table 194. Hematology: fasting baseline, men and women aged 60–69 years (7:00–9:00 A.M.)

	n	Mean	SD	CI-Up.	CI-Lo.	Med.	Max.	Min.	Lo.Qt.	Up.Qt.	RR-Lo.L	RR-Up.L
Leukocytes (10^9/l)	603	6.54	1.46	6.66	6.43	6.1	12.5	4.4	5.6	7.1	4.8	10.4
Erythrocytes (10^{12}/l)	603	4.63	0.39	4.66	4.60	4.62	5.74	3.8	4.33	4.95	3.94	5.41
Hemoglobin (g/dl)	603	14.03	1.37	14.14	13.92	14.1	17.6	10.3	13.1	15.0	11.3	16.4
Hematocrit (%)	547	42.26	3.77	42.57	41.94	42.4	52.1	33.0	39.6	44.9	34.3	49.4
MCV (fl)	548	90.63	4.49	91.01	90.26	90.6	109.9	72.8	88.4	93.6	81.6	98.4
MCH (pg/cell)	498	30.30	1.75	30.46	30.15	30.4	37.8	22.0	29.4	31.4	25.8	33.3
MCHC (g Hb/dl Er.)	548	33.52	1.17	33.61	33.42	33.5	36.8	30.8	32.8	34.3	31.4	35.7
Platelets (thrombocytes; 10^9/l)	602	252.07	62.66	257.08	247.07	241	524	142	205	276	155	325
Lymphocytes (%)	600	32.87	7.76	33.49	32.25	32	56	10	27	38	20	49
Monocytes (%)	603	3.72	2.35	3.91	3.54	4	10	0	2	5	0	9
Eosinophils (%)	603	2.69	1.82	2.83	2.54	2	13	0	1	4	0	7
Basophils (%)	603	0.56	0.66	0.61	0.51	0	4	0	0	1	0	2
Segmented neutrophils (%)	599	60.01	8.01	60.65	59.36	61	80	37	55	66	44	74
Bands (%)	427	0.07	0.33	0.11	0.04	0	3	0	0	0	0	1
Reticulocytes (‰)	209	14.37	5.74	15.15	13.60	13	31	0	10	17	6	28
Quick's test (%)	537	113.36	12.22	114.39	112.33	113	152	82	105	121	91	138
Age (years)	603	66.2	2.8	–	–	–	69	60	–	–	–	–

SD, Standard deviation; *CI-Up.*, 95% upper confidence limit; *CI-Lo*, 95% lower confidence limit; *Med*, median; *Max*, maximum; *Min.*, minimum; *Lo.Q*, lower quartile; *Up.Qt*, upper quarter; *RR-Lo.L*, lower limit of reference range; *RR-Up.L*, upper limit of reference range; *MCV*, mean corpuscular volume; *MCH*, mean corpuscular hemoglobin; *MCHC*, mean corpuscular hemoglobin concentration.

Table 195. Hematology: fasting baseline, men and women aged 70–80 years (7:00–9:00 A.M.)

	n	Mean	SD	CI-Up.	CI-Lo.	Med.	Max.	Min.	Lo.Qt.	Up.Qt.	RR-Lo.L	RR-Up.L
Leukocytes (10^9/l)	177	6.26	1.09	6.42	6.10	6.0	10.9	4.4	5.6	6.7	5.0	9.4
Erythrocytes (10^{12}/l)	177	4.55	0.37	4.61	4.50	4.6	5.4	3.7	4.3	4.9	3.9	5.3
Hemoglobin (g/dl)	177	13.71	1.24	13.89	13.52	13.7	16.5	10.9	12.9	14.5	11.4	16.2
Hematocrit (%)	173	40.84	3.72	41.39	40.28	40.2	51.6	31.7	38.1	43.6	34.4	48.7
MCV (fl)	173	89.81	4.58	90.50	89.13	90.5	100.0	71.1	87.2	92.7	80.0	97.7
MCH (pg/cell)	156	30.10	1.97	30.41	29.79	30.7	34.0	22.4	29.0	31.5	25.6	32.9
MCHC (g Hb/dl Er.)	173	33.67	1.04	33.83	33.52	33.7	36.4	30.9	32.9	34.5	31.5	35.6
Platelets (thrombocytes; 10^9/l)	176	250.01	71.11	260.51	239.50	230	519	144	198	297	153	467
Lymphocytes (%)	174	34.41	7.96	35.59	33.23	34	54	15	30	40	19	54
Monocytes (%)	177	3.71	2.81	4.13	3.30	3	11	0	2	5	0	10
Eosinophils (%)	177	2.98	2.09	3.29	2.67	3	11	0	1	4	0	9
Basophils (%)	177	0.47	0.63	0.57	0.38	0	3	0	0	1	0	2
Segmented neutrophils (%)	174	58.20	8.19	59.41	56.98	58	85	33	52	64	44	85
Bands (%)	162	0.04	0.23	0.08	0.01	0	2	0	0	0	0	1
Reticulocytes (‰)	68	12.99	4.26	14.00	11.97	13	24	5	10	16	6	24
Quick's test (%)	170	112.31	10.60	113.91	110.72	111	139	83	106	120	92	139
Age (years)	177	75.4	2.5	–	–	–	80	70	–	–	–	–

SD, Standard deviation; *CI-Up.*, 95% upper confidence limit; *CI-Lo*, 95% lower confidence limit; *Med*, median; *Max*, maximum; *Min.*, minimum; *Lo.Q.*, lower quartile; *Up.Qt.*, upper quarter; *RR-Lo.L*, lower limit of reference range; *RR-Up.L*, upper limit of reference range; *MCV*, mean corpuscular volume; *MCH*, mean corpuscular hemoglobin; *MCHC*, mean corpuscular hemoglobin concentration.

6.7.1.2 Young Subjects

Table 196. Hematology: fasting baseline, men aged 20–39 years (7:00–9:00 A.M.)

	n	Mean	SD	CI-Up.	CI-Lo.	Med.	Max.	Min.	Lo.Qt.	Up.Qt.	RR-Lo.L	RR-Up.L
Leukocytes (10^9/l)	1434	6.47	1.63	6.56	6.39	6.2	14.6	4.0	5.2	7.3	4.3	10.7
Erythrocytes (10^{12}/l)	1445	4.91	0.36	4.92	4.89	4.89	8.4	4.2	4.65	5.13	4.28	5.60
Hemoglobin (g/dl)	1482	14.87	1.04	14.93	14.82	14.9	17.9	12.4	14.2	15.6	12.8	16.9
Hematocrit (%)	1492	43.98	3.33	44.15	43.81	44.0	55.7	35.8	41.7	46.1	37.6	50.4
MCV (fl)	1496	90.45	4.38	90.68	90.23	90.2	109.2	78.9	87.4	93.2	82.7	99.9
MCHC (g Hb/dl Er.)	1501	33.89	1.23	33.95	33.82	33.9	37.7	28.7	33.1	34.7	31.5	36.3
Platelets (thrombocytes; 10^9/l)	1415	239.73	45.08	242.08	237.38	234	461	164	207	266.0	170.0	343.0
Lymphocytes (%)	1397	38.26	7.94	38.67	37.84	38	77	23	32	43	25	55
Monocytes (%)	1451	3.73	2.58	3.87	3.60	4	11	0	2	6	0	9
Eosinophils (%)	1451	3.14	2.19	3.26	3.03	3	17	0	2	4	0	8
Basophils (%)	1386	0.58	0.73	0.61	0.54	0	5	0	0	1	0	2
Segmented neutrophils (%)	1087	55.09	8.36	55.59	54.59	55	82	35	50	61	39	72
Bands (%)	1118	0.06	0.31	0.08	0.04	0	4	0	0	0	0	1
Quick's test (%)	1387	104.65	12.00	105.29	104.02	104	145	70	97	112	82	130
Age (years)	1522	27.2	3.8	–	–	–	39	20	–	–	–	–

SD, Standard deviation; *CI-Up.*, 95% upper confidence limit; *CI-Lo.*, 95% lower confidence limit; *Med.*, median; *Min.*, minimum; *Lo.Q.*, lower quartile; *Up.Qt.*, upper quarter; *RR-Lo.L*, lower limit of reference range; *RR-Up.L*, upper limit of reference range; *MCH*, mean corpuscular hemoglobin; *MCHC*, mean corpuscular hemoglobin concentration.

Table 197. Hematology: fasting baseline, men aged 20–29 years (7:00–9:00 A.M.)

	n	Mean	SD	CI-Up.	CI-Lo.	Med.	Max.	Min.	Lo.Qt.	Up.Qt.	RR-Lo.L	RR-Up.L
Leukocytes (10^9/l)	1123	6.39	1.54	6.48	6.30	6.1	14.5	4.0	5.2	7.2	4.3	10.6
Erythrocytes (10^{12}/l)	1138	4.92	0.36	4.94	4.90	4.91	8.40	4.20	4.66	5.14	4.28	5.60
Hemoglobin (g/dl)	1156	14.92	1.02	14.98	14.86	15.0	17.9	12.4	14.2	15.6	12.8	16.8
Hematocrit (%)	1164	44.12	3.30	44.31	43.93	44.2	55.7	35.8	41.9	46.2	37.6	50.5
MCV (fl)	1168	90.35	4.47	90.61	90.10	90.0	109.2	78.9	87.4	93.0	82.2	100.2
MCHC (g Hb/dl Er.)	1173	33.89	1.23	33.96	33.82	33.9	37.7	28.7	33.1	34.7	31.4	36.3
Platelets (thrombocytes; 10^9/l)	1104	239.58	45.54	242.26	236.89	235	461	164	207	267	170	342.0
Lymphocytes (%)	1090	38.44	7.85	38.90	37.97	38	70	23	33	43	25	55
Monocytes (%)	1133	3.63	2.63	3.79	3.48	4	11	0	1	6	0	9
Eosinophils (%)	1133	3.03	2.09	3.15	2.91	3	17	0	2	4	0	8
Basophils (%)	1092	0.59	0.74	0.63	0.54	0	5	0	0	1	0	2
Segmented neutrophils (%)	865	55.17	8.47	55.74	54.61	55	82	35	50	61	39	72
Bands (%)	889	0.06	0.33	0.08	0.04	0	4	0	0	0	0	1
Quick's test (%)	1100	104.50	12.17	105.21	103.78	104	144	70	96	112	82	130
Age (years)	1193	25.7	2.4	–	–	–	29	20	–	–	–	–

SD, Standard deviation; *CI-Up.*, 95% upper confidence limit; *CI-Lo.*, 95% lower confidence limit; *Med.*, median; *Max.*, maximum; *Min.*, minimum; *Lo.Q.*, lower quartile; *Up.Qt.*, upper quarter; *RR-Lo.L*, lower limit of reference range; *RR-Up.L*, upper limit of reference range; *MCH*, mean corpuscular hemoglobin; *MCHC*, mean corpuscular hemoglobin concentration.

Table 198. Hematology: fasting baseline, men aged 30–39 years (7:00–9:00 A.M.)

	n	Mean	SD	CI-Up.	CI-Lo.	Med.	Max.	Min.	Lo.Qt.	Up.Qt.	RR-Lo.L	RR-Up.L
Leukocytes (10⁹/l)	311	6.78	1.91	6.99	6.57	6.5	14.6	4.1	5.2	7.9	4.3	11.5
Erythrocytes 10¹²/l)	307	4.86	0.36	4.90	4.82	4.84	7.00	4.21	4.59	5.09	4.33	5.58
Hemoglobin (g/dl)	326	14.72	1.09	14.84	14.61	14.7	17.7	12.5	13.9	15.4	12.7	17.1
Hematocrit (%)	328	43.48	3.41	43.85	43.11	43.5	53.0	35.9	41.0	45.7	37.0	49.9
MCV (fl)	328	90.82	4.03	91.25	90.38	90.7	100.6	82.0	87.9	93.7	83.1	99.1
MCHC (g Hb/dl Er.)	328	33.89	1.26	34.02	33.75	33.9	36.9	29.0	32.9	34.8	31.7	36.5
Platelets (thrombocytes; 10⁹/l)	311	240.25	43.51	245.09	235.42	233	434	166	208	265	176	352
Lymphocytes (%)	307	37.62	8.22	38.54	36.70	36	77	23	32	43	25	55
Monocytes (%)	318	4.10	2.37	4.36	3.84	4	10	0	2	6	0	9
Eosinophils (%)	318	3.55	2.46	3.82	3.28	3	14	0	2	5	0	9
Basophils (%)	294	0.54	0.69	0.62	0.46	0	3	0	0	1	0	2
Segmented neutrophils (%)	222	54.77	7.93	55.81	53.72	55	79	35	50	61	40	69
Bands (%)	229	0.04	0.23	0.07	0.01	0	2	0	0	0	0	1
Quick's test (%)	287	105.26	11.29	106.57	103.96	105	145	71	100	112	82	132
Age (years)	329	32.8	2.3	–	–	–	39	30	–	–	–	–

SD, Standard deviation; *CI-Up.*, 95% upper confidence limit; *CI-Lo*, 95% lower confidence limit; *Med.*, median; *Max.*, maximum; *Min.*, minimum; *Lo.Q.*, lower quartile; *Up.Qt.*, upper quarter; *RR-Lo.L*, lower limit of reference range; *RR-Up.L*, upper limit of reference range; *MCV*, mean corpuscular volume; *MCH*, mean corpuscular hemoglobin; *MCHC*, mean corpuscular hemoglobin concentration.

6.7.2 Changes After Repeated Measurements

Table 199. Hematology: changes after 24 h, differences from baseline, men and women aged 50–80 years (7:00–9:00 A.M.)

	n	Mean	SD	CI-Up.	CI-Lo.	Med.	Max.	Min.	Lo.Qt.	Up.Qt.	RR-Lo.L	RR-Up.L	D_crit
Leukocytes (10^9/l)	211	-0.02	0.98	0.12	-0.15	0.0	3.2	-3.3	-0.6	0.6	-2.2	2.1	2.10
Erythrocytes (10^{12}/l)	211	-0.09	0.24	-0.06	-0.13	-0.07	0.52	-1.04	-0.22	0.05	-0.63	0.40	0.46
Hemoglobin	211	-0.33	0.80	-0.22	-0.44	-0.2	1.3	-3.2	-0.6	0.1	-2.5	1.0	1.55
Hematocrit (%)	211	-0.89	2.10	-0.61	-1.17	-0.7	4.3	-8.0	-2.0	0.4	-6.0	3.2	4.08
MCH (pg/cell)	200	-0.08	0.94	0.05	-0.21	0.0	2.6	-3.5	-0.4	0.4	-2.9	1.7	1.73
MCV (fl)	199	0.05	1.78	0.29	-0.20	-0.1	13.0	-6.8	-0.7	0.8	-2.8	3.8	3.47
MCHC (g Hb/dl Er.)	152	0.12	1.08	0.30	-0.05	0.1	4.3	-6.7	-0.3	0.6	-1.9	2.1	2.05
Platelets	211	-2.68	27.61	1.05	-6.40	-2	98	-86	-14	12	-83	56	53.67
Lymphocytes (%)	200	0.97	5.74	1.76	0.17	1	15	-13	-3	5	-10	12	11.08
Monocytes (%)	211	0.37	1.99	0.64	0.11	0	6	-4	-1	2	-3	5	3.53
Basophils (%)	163	-0.01	0.92	0.13	-0.15	0	3	-3	-1	0	-2	2	1.79
Eosinophils (%)	211	0.10	1.42	0.29	-0.09	0	7	-5	-1	1	-3	3	2.06
Bands (%)	114	0.01	0.34	0.07	-0.05	0	2	-1	0	0	-1	1	0.58
Segmented neutrophils (%)	211	-0.88	7.15	0.08	-1.85	-1	23	-19	-5	3	-15	17	8.24
Reticulocytes (‰)	114	1.49	4.64	2.34	0.64	1	24	-8	-1	4	-5	14	12.44
Quick's test (%)	200	-0.27	7.20	0.73	-1.26	0	15	-37	-4	4	-12	12	13.17
Age (years)	211	67.6	6.0	–	–	–	80	51	–	–	–	–	–

SD, Standard deviation; *CI-Up.*, 95% upper confidence limit; *CI-Lo.*, 95% lower confidence limit; *Med.*, median; *Max.*, maximum; *Min.*, minimum; *Lo.Q.*, lower quartile; *Up.Qt.*, upper quarter; *RR-Lo.L*, lower limit of reference range; *RR-Up.L*, upper limit of reference range; *MCV*, mean corpuscular volume; *MCH*, mean corpuscular hemoglobin; *MCHC*, mean corpuscular hemoglobin concentration; D_{crit}, critical difference 0.05.

Table 200. Hematology: changes after 1 week, differences from baseline, men and women aged 50–80 years (7:00–9:00 A.M.)

	n	Mean	SD	CI-Up.	CI-Lo.	Med.	Max.	Min.	Lo.Qt.	Up.Qt.	RR-Lo.L	RR-Up.L	D_{crit}
Leukocytes (10^9/l)	240	-0.02	0.89	0.09	-0.13	0.0	2.5	-2.1	-0.6	0.6	-1.9	1.9	1.75
Erythrocytes (10^{12}/l)	240	-0.02	0.20	0.00	-0.05	0.00	0.52	-0.64	-0.14	0.11	-0.42	0.32	0.39
Hemoglobin	240	-0.10	0.57	-0.03	-0.18	-0.1	1.5	-1.9	-0.4	0.3	-1.2	1.1	1.11
Hematocrit (%)	240	-0.44	2.07	-0.18	-0.71	-0.4	5.4	-10.7	-1.8	1.0	-4.4	3.3	4.01
MCH (pg/cell)	230	-0.30	1.51	-0.10	-0.49	-0.2	6.3	-6.8	-1.1	0.4	-3.3	2.9	2.88
MCV (fl)	219	-0.02	0.62	0.06	-0.11	-0.1	2.6	-1.9	-0.4	0.3	-1.3	1.5	1.22
MCHC (g Hb/dl Er.)	230	0.12	1.04	0.25	-0.02	0.1	7.1	-3.8	-0.4	0.6	-2.2	2.0	2.02
Platelets	240	4.35	20.96	7.00	1.69	4	54	-56	-10	19	-37	48	40.65
Lymphocytes (%)	218	-0.22	5.66	0.54	-0.97	0	14	-15	-4	4	-13	10	10.33
Monocytes (%)	240	-0.13	1.87	0.10	-0.37	0	5	-4	-2	1	-4	4	3.53
Basophils (%)	240	0.00	0.90	0.11	-0.11	0	3	-3	-1	1	-1	2	1.67
Eosinophils (%)	240	0.03	1.75	0.25	-0.20	0	6	-7	-1	1	-4	3	3.43
Bands (%)	230	0.13	5.43	0.84	-0.57	0	13	-13	-4	4	-10	10	9.90
Segmented neutrophils (%)	179	0.03	0.47	0.10	-0.04	0	3	-3	0	0	-1	1	0.84
Reticulocytes (‰)	159	1.41	4.86	2.16	0.65	1	13	-11	-2	5	-8	12	9.45
Quick's test (%)	230	0.94	8.05	1.98	-0.10	1	22	-19	-5	6	-14	16	15.30
Age (years)	240	67.0	5.9	–	–	–	80	50	–	–	–	–	–

SD, Standard deviation; *CI-Up.*, 95% upper confidence limit; *CI-Lo.*, 95% lower confidence limit; *Med.*, median; *Max.*, maximum; *Min.*, minimum; *Lo.Q.*, lower quartile; *Up.Qt.*, upper quarter; *RR-Lo.L*, lower limit of reference range; *RR-Up.L*, upper limit of reference range; *MCV*, mean corpuscular volume; *MCH*, mean corpuscular hemoglobin; *MCHC*, mean corpuscular hemoglobin concentration; *D_{crit}*, critical difference 0.05.

Table 201. Hematology: changes after 2 weeks, differences from baseline, men and women aged 50–80 years (7:00–9:00 A.M.)

	n	Mean	SD	CI-Up.	CI-Lo.	Med.	Max.	Min.	Lo.Qt.	Up.Qt.	RR-Lo.L	RR-Up.L	D_crit
Leukocytes (10^9/l)	225	-0.16	0.82	-0.05	-0.27	-0.1	1.9	-2.2	-0.7	0.4	-1.7	1.5	1.75
Erythrocytes (10^{12}/l)	225	-0.06	0.22	-0.03	-0.09	-0.04	0.59	-1.1	-0.19	0.07	-0.53	0.33	0.43
Hemoglobin	225	-0.22	0.62	-0.14	-0.30	-0.2	1.4	-2.1	-0.6	0.2	-1.5	1	1.21
Hematocrit (%)	225	-0.60	2.14	-0.32	-0.88	-0.4	11.8	-6	-1.9	0.7	-4.6	2.8	4.14
MCH (pg/cell)	215	-0.24	1.36	-0.06	-0.42	-0.2	5.4	-3.4	-1.2	0.5	-2.8	3	2.66
MCV (fl)	215	-0.08	0.66	0.01	-0.16	-0.1	2.3	-2.4	-0.5	0.3	-1.1	1.4	1.24
MCHC (g Hb/dl Er.)	215	0.01	0.78	0.12	-0.09	-0.1	3.5	-3.4	-0.5	0.4	-1.3	1.8	1.48
Platelets	225	5.28	18.69	7.73	2.84	7	61	-48	-8	17	-31	39	45.17
Lymphocytes (%)	199	-1.09	6.17	-0.23	-1.94	-1	15	-18	-5	3	-14	11	12.4
Monocytes (%)	225	-0.03	2.34	0.28	-0.33	0	5	-7	-1	1	-5	5	4.23
Basophils (%)	225	-0.06	0.93	0.06	-0.18	0	3	-3	-1	0	-2	2	1.79
Eosinophils (%)	225	-0.11	1.94	0.15	-0.36	0	6	-7	-1	1	-4	5	3.66
Bands (%)	211	0.92	5.46	1.66	0.19	1	12	-13	-4	5	-9	10	12.76
Segmented neutrophils (%)	195	0.02	0.39	0.07	-0.04	0	2	-3	0	0	-1	1	0.74
Reticulocytes (‰)	135	1.47	4.88	2.29	0.64	2	16	-10	-2	5	-8	11	10.98
Quick's test (%)	211	1.37	8.08	2.46	0.28	2	21	-17	-4	7	-15	17	14.57
Age (years)	225	66.9	6.1	-	-	-	80	50	-	-	-	-	-

SD, Standard deviation; *CI-Up.*, 95% upper confidence limit; *CI-Lo.*, 95% lower confidence limit; *Med.*, median; *Max.*, maximum; *Min.*, minimum; *Lo.Q.*, lower quartile; *Up.Qt.*, upper quarter; *RR-Lo.L*, lower limit of reference range; *RR-Up.L*, upper limit of reference range; *MCH*, mean corpuscular hemoglobin; *MCHC*, mean corpuscular hemoglobin concentration; *MCV*, mean corpuscular volume; *D_crit*, critical difference 0.05.

Table 202. Hematology: changes after 3 weeks, differences from baseline, men and women aged 50–80 years (7:00–9:00 A.M.)

	n	Mean	SD	CI-Up.	CI-Lo.	Med.	Max.	Min.	Lo.Qt.	Up.Qt.	RR-Lo.L	RR-Up.L	D$_{crit}$
Leukocytes (10^9/l)	172	-0.26	0.85	-0.13	-0.39	-0.4	2.2	-1.9	-0.9	0.3	-1.7	1.6	1.60
Erythrocytes (10^{12}/l)	172	-0.06	0.24	-0.03	-0.10	-0.08	0.63	-0.79	-0.19	0.10	-0.60	0.54	0.47
Hemoglobin	172	-0.22	0.59	-0.13	-0.31	-0.3	1.6	-1.4	-0.6	0.1	-1.3	1.3	1.15
Hematocrit (%)	172	-0.74	2.92	-0.30	-1.18	-1.0	8.8	-10.0	-2.2	0.9	-6.9	5.8	5.62
MCH (pg/cell)	162	-0.19	2.93	0.26	-0.64	-0.5	14.1	-9.4	-1.5	0.7	-4.4	7.8	5.45
MCV (fl)	162	-0.14	1.14	0.04	-0.31	-0.2	5.2	-4.8	-0.6	0.4	-2.3	3.4	2.19
MCHC (g Hb/dl Er.)	162	-0.07	1.23	0.12	-0.26	-0.1	4.8	-5.3	-0.5	0.6	-2.3	2.1	1.81
Platelets	172	1.53	24.13	5.14	-2.07	-1	66	-50	-15	18	-44	50	46.28
Lymphocytes (%)	172	-0.57	8.46	0.69	-1.83	0	27	-21	-6	4	-17	17	15.98
Monocytes (%)	172	-0.07	2.67	0.33	-0.47	0	6	-8	-1	2	-6	6	5.04
Basophils (%)	172	0.03	0.92	0.17	-0.10	0	2	-3	0	1	-2	2	1.26
Eosinophils (%)	172	0.07	2.16	0.39	-0.25	0	9	-8	-1	1	-4	5	4.09
Bands (%)	172	0.72	9.03	2.07	-0.63	0	28	-22	-4	7	-18	20	17.57
Segmented neutrophils (%)	162	0.07	0.59	0.16	-0.02	0	6	-1	0	0	-1	1	0.49
Reticulocytes (‰)	138	1.24	4.85	2.05	0.43	2	12	-11	-2	5	-8	10	9.18
Quick's test (%)	162	1.10	9.97	2.64	-0.43	1	34	-30	-5	7	-18	24	19.44
Age (years)	172	66.39	5.82	–	–	–	80	51	–	–	–	–	–

SD, Standard deviation; *CI-Up.*, 95% upper confidence limit; *CI-Lo.*, 95% lower confidence limit; *Med.*, median; *Max.*, maximum; *Min.*, minimum; *Lo.Q.*, lower quartile; *Up.Qt.*, upper quarter; *RR-Lo.L*, lower limit of reference range; *RR-Up.L*, upper limit of reference range; *MCV*, mean corpuscular volume; *MCH*, mean corpuscular hemoglobin; *MCHC*, mean corpuscular hemoglobin concentration; *D$_{crit}$* critical difference 0.05.

References

Adams KRH, Martin JA (1991) Electrolyte disorders in the elderly. Drugs Aging 1 (4):254–265

Anders TR, Fozard JL (1973) Effects of age upon retrieval from primary and secondary memory. Dev Psychol 6:214–217

Bach B, Hansen JM, Kampmann JP, Rasmussen SN, Skovsted L (1981) Disposition of antipyrine and phenytoin correlated with age and liver volume in man. Clin Pharmacokinet 6:389–396

Baddeley A (1986) Working memory. Clarendon, Oxford

Barlett HL, Puhl SM, Hodgson JL, Buskirk ER (1991) Fat-free mass in relation to stature: ratios of fat-free mass to height in children, adults, and elderly subjects. Am J Clin Nutr 53:1112–1116

Barnes RH, Busse EW, Friedland EL (1956) The psychological function of aged individuals with normal and abnormal electroencephalograms. II. A study of hospitalized individuals. J Nerv Ment Dis 124:585–593

Bauer JH (1993) Age-related changes in the renin-aldosterone system. Physiological effects and clinical implications. Drugs Aging 3 (3):238–245

Bellville JW, Forrest WH, Miller E, Brown BW (1971) Influence of age on pain relief from analgesics. A study of postoperative patients. J Am Med Assoc 217:1835–1841

Bender AD (1968) Effect of age on intestinal absorption: implications for drug asorption in the elderly. J Am Geriatr Soc 16:1331–1339

Bertel O, Landemann R, Lutold BE, Bolli P (1980) Plasma catecholamines and cardiac renal and peripheral vascular adrenoceptor mediated responses in different age groups in normal and hypertensive subjects. Clin Exp Hypertens 2:409–426

Besa EC (1988) Approach to mild anemia in the elderly. Clin Geriatr Med 4:43–55

Bethge KP, Bethge D, Meiners G, Lichtlen PR (1983) Incidence and prognostic significance of ventricular arrhythmias in individuals without detectable heart disease. Eur Heart J 4 (5):338–346

Bjerregaard P (1982) Premature beats in healthy subjects 40–79 years of age. Eur Heart J 3 (6):493–503

Bjorksten J (1971) The crosslinkage theory of aging. Finska Kemists Med 80(2):23

Bleich HL, Boro ES, Rowe JW (1977) Clinical research on aging: strategies and directions. N Engl J Med 297 (24):1332–1336

Bondareff, W (1977) The neural basis of aging. In: Birren JE, Schaie KW (eds) Handbook of the psychology of aging. Van Nostrand Reinhold, New York, pp 157–176

Bottiger LE, Svedberg CA (1967) Normal erythrocyte sedimentation rate and age. BMJ 2:85–87

Boyd JC, Lacher DA (1982) The multivariate reference range: an alternative interpretation of multi-test profiles. Clin Chem 28 (2):259–265

Brandfonbrener M, Landowne M, Shock NW (1955) Changes in cardiac output with age. Circulation 12:557

Brizzee KR, Ordy JM, Kaack B (1974) Early appearance and regional differences in intraneuronal and extraneuronal lipofuscin accumulation with age in the brain of a nonhuman primate (Macaca mulatta). J Gerontol 29:366–381

Brodsky M, Wu D, Denes P, Kanakis C, Rosen KM (1977) Arrhythmias documented by 24 hour continuous electrocardiographic monitoring in 50 male medical students without apparent heart disease. Am J Cardiol 39 (3):390–395

Brody H (1973) Aging of the vertebrate brain. In: Rockstein M (ed) Development and aging in the nervous system. Academic, New York, pp 123–153

Busse EW, Barnes RH, Silverman AJ, Shy GM, Thaler M, Frost LL (1954) Studies of the process of aging: factors that influence the psyche of elderly persons. Am J Psychiatry 110:897–903

Busse EW, Barnes RH, Friedman EL, Kelty EJ (1956) Psychological functioning of aged individuals with normal and abnormal electroencephalograms. I. A study of non-hospitalized community volunteers. J Nerv Ment Dis 12 4:135–141

Byyny RL (1990) Hypertension in the elderly. In: Laragh JH, Brenner D (eds) Hypertension: pathophysiology, diagnosis, and management. Raven, New York, pp 1869–1887

Caird FI, Scott PJW (1986) Drug induced diseases in the elderly. Elsevier, Amsterdam

Calloway NO, Foley CF, Lagerbloom P (1965) Uncertainties in geriatric data. II. Organ size. J Am Geriatr Soc 13:20–28

Campion EW, deLabry LO, Glynn RJ (1988) The effect of age on serum albumin in healthy males; report from the normative aging study. J Gernontol 43M:18–20

Castleden CM, George CF, Marcer D, Hallett C (1977) Increased sensitivity to nitrazepam in old age. BMJ 1:10–12

Castleden CM, George CF (1979) The effect of ageing on the hepatic clearance of propranolol. Br J Clin Pharmacol 7:49–54

Cattell RB (1971) Abilities: their structure, growth, and action. Houghton, Boston

Chandler MHH, Scott SR, Blouin RA (1988) Age-associated stereoselective alterations in hexobarbital metabolism. Clin Pharmacol Ther 43:436–441

Christian W (1984) Das Elektroencephalogramm (EEG) im höheren Lebensalter. Nervenarzt 55:517–524

Clark WC, Mehl L (1971) Thermal pain: a sensory decision theory analysis of the effect of age and sex on d', various response criteria, and 50 percent pain threshold. J Abnorm Psychol 78:202–212

Cody RJ (1993) Physiological changes due to age, implications for drug therapy of congestive heart failure. Drugs Aging 3 (4):320–334

Conway J, Wheeler R, Sannerstedt R (1971) Sympathetic nervous activity during exercise in relation to age. Cardiovasc Res 5:577–581

Corberand J, Laharrague P, Fillola G (1987) Blood cell parameters do not change during physiological human ageing. Gerontology 33:72–76

Costongs GMPJ, Janson PCW (1984) Effects of biological and analytical variations on the appropriate use of "reference intervals" in clinical chemistry. Proposal of a scheme for longitudinal assessment of laboratory values. J Clin Chem Clin Biochem 22:613–621

Costongs GMPJ, Janson PCW, Brombacher PJ (1984) Effects of biological and analytical variations on the approprate use of age on hematopoiesis in man. Blood 63:502–509

Costongs GMPJ, Bas BM, Janson PCW, Hermans J, Brombacher PJ, van Wersch JWJ (1985a) Short-term and long-term intra-individual variations and critical differences of coagulation parameters. J Clin Chem Clin Biochem 23:405–410

Costongs GMPJ, Janson PCW, Bas B, Hermans J, van Wersch JWJ, Brombacher PJ (1985b) Short-term and long-term intra-individual variations and critical differences of clinical chemical laboratory parameters. J Clin Chem Clin Biochem 23:7–16

Costongs GMPJ, Janson PCW, Bas BM, Hermans J, van Wersch JWJ, Brombacher PJ (1985c) Short-term and long-term intra-individual variations and critical differences of hematological laboratory parameters. J Clin Chem Clin Biochem 23:69–76

Cox J, O'Malley K, Atkins N, O'Brien E (1991) A comparision of the twenty-four-hour blood pressure profile in normotensive and hypertensive subjects. J Hypertens 9 (1):3–6

Craik FLM (1977) Age differences in human memory. In: Birren JE, Schaie KW (eds) Handbook of the psychology of aging. Van Nostrand Reinhold, New York, pp 384–420

Craik IFM (1968) Short-term memory and the aging process. Talland GA (ed) Human aging and behavior. Academic, New York, pp 131–168

Critchley M (1942) Ageing of the nervous system. In: Cowdry EV (ed) Problems of ageing. Williams and Wilkins, Baltimore, pp 518–534

Crooks J (1983) Aging and drug disposition: pharmacodynamics. J Chronic Dis 36:85–90

Culver BH, Butler J (1985) Alterations in pulmonary functions. In: Andres R et al (eds) Principles of geriatric medicine. McGraw-Hill, New York, pp 280–287

Curran, S (1991) Critical flicker fusion in gertonological research: clinical implications for Alzheimer's disease. In: Hindmarch I, Hippius H, Wilcock GK (eds) Dementia: molecules, methods and measures. Wiley, Chichester, pp 169–176

Davies DF, Shock NW (1950) Age changes in glomerular filtration rate, efective renal plasma flow, and tubular excretory capacity in adult males. J Clin Invest 29:496–507

Davies I (1985) Biology of aging – theories of aging. In: Brockehurst JC (ed) Textbook of eriatric medicine and gerontology, 3rd edn. Churchill Livingstone, New York

Davies P (1979) Neurotransmitter-related enzymes in senile dementia of the Alzheimer type. Brain Res 171:319–327

Dehn MM, Bruce RA (1971) Longitudinal variations in maximal oxygen intake with age and activity. J Appl Physiol 33:805

DeLeon MJ, Ferris SH, George AE, Reisberg B, Christman D, Kritcheff II, Wolf AP (1983) Computed tomography and positron emission transaxial tomography evaluations of normal aging and Alzheimer's disease. J Cereb Blood Flow Metab 3:391–394

Docherty JR (1986) Aging and the cardiovascular system. J Auton Pharmacol 6:77–84

Duffy FH, Albert MS, McAnulty G (1984) Brain electrical activity in patients with presenile and senile dementia of the Alzheimer type. Ann Neurol 16:439–448

Durnas C, Loi C-M, Cusack BJ (1990) Hepatic drug metabolism and aging. Clini Pharmacokinet 1 (5):359–389

Dybkaer R, Lauritzen M, Krakauer R (1981) Relative reference values for clinical chemical and haematological quantities in 'healthy' elderly people. Acta Med Scand 209:1–9

Ebersole P, Hess P (1990) Toward healthy aging: human needs and nursing response, 3rd edn. Mosby, St Louis

Eisdorfer C (1968) Arousal and performance: experiments in verbal learning and a tentative theory. In: Talland GA (ed) Human aging and behavior. Academic, New York, pp 189–216

Engen T (1977) Taste and smell. In: Birren JE, Schaie KW (eds) Handbook of the psychology aging. Van Nostrand Reinhold, New York, pp 554–561

Feinberg I (1969) Effects of age on human sleep patterns. In: Kales A (ed) Sleep physiology and pathology. Lippincott, Philadelphia, pp 39–52

Feldman R, Limbird LE, Nadeau J, Fitzgerald GA, Robertson D et al (1983) Dynamic regulations of leukocyte beta-adrenergic receptor-agonist interactions by physiological changes in circulating catecholamines. J Clin Invest 72:164–170

Feldman RD, Limbird LE, Nadeau J, Fitzgerald GA, Wood AJJ (1984) Alterations in leukocyte beta-receptor affinity with aging: a potential explanation for altered beta-adrenergic sensitivity in the elderly. N Engl J Med 310:815–819

Ferszt R, Gertz HJ (1982) Morphologie des physiologischen Alterns und des hirnorganischen Psychosyndroms. In: Bente D, Coper H, Kanowski S (eds) Hirnorganische Psychosyndrome im Alter. Springer, Berlin Heidelberg New York, pp 123–153

Fleg JL, Kennedy HL (1982) Cardiac arrhythmias in a healthy elderly population. Detection by 24 hour ambulatroy electrocardiography. Chest 81:302

Fleg JL, Tzankoff SP, Lakatta EG (1985) Age-related augmentation of plasma catecholamines during dynamic exercise in healthy males. J Appl Physiol 59:1033–1039

Fletcher GF, Froelicher VF, Hartley LH, Haskell WL, Pollock ML (1990) Exercise standards. A statement for health professionals form the American Heart Association. Circulation 82:2286–2322

Food and Drug Administration, Center for Drug Evaluation, Department of Health and Human Services, Public Health Service (1989) Guideline for the study of drugs likely to be used in the elderly

Forette F, McClaran J, Herry MP, Bouchacourt P, Henry JF (1989) Nicardipine in elderly patients with hypertension: a review of experience in France. Am Heart J 117:256–261

Fozard JL, Wolf E, Bell B, McFarland RA, Podolsky S (1977) Visual perception and communication. In: Birren JE, Schaie KW (eds) Handbook of the psychology of aging. Van Nostrand Reinhold, New York, pp 497–534

Frackowiak RSJ, Lenzi GL, Jones T, Heather JD (1980) Quantitative measurement of regional cerebral blood flow and oxygen metabolism in man using 15 O and positron emission tomography: theory, procedure, and normal values. J Comp Assist Tomogr 4:727–736

Fraser CG (1993) Age-related changes in laboratory test results. Clinical implications. Drugs Aging 3 (3):246–257

Fraser CG, Fogarty Y (1989) Interpreting laboratory results. BMJ 298 (6689):1659–1660

Fraser CG, Cummings ST, Wilkinson SP, Neville RG, Knox JDE, Ho O, MacWalter RS (1989a) Biological variability of 26 clinical chemistry analytes in elderly people. Clin Chem 35 (5):783–786

Fraser CG, Wilkinson SP, Nevill RG, Knox JDE, King JF, McWalter RS (1989b) Biologic variation of common hematologic laboratory quantities in the elderly. Am J Clin Pathol 92:465–470

Gerstenblith G, Frederiksen J, Yin FCP et al (1977) Echocardiographic assessment of a normal adult aging population. Circulation 56:273

Gibbs FA, Gibbs EL (1950) Atlas of encephalography, vol 1. Methodology and controls. Addison-Wesley, Cambridge

Gilbertson VA (1965) Erythrocyte sedimentation rates in older patients: a study of 4341 cases. Postgrad Med 38:A44–52

Goff GB, Rosner BS, Detre T, Kennard D (1965) Vibration perception in normal man and medical patients. J Neurol Neurosurg Psychiatry 28:503

Grahame-Smith DJ, Aronson JK (1984) The Oxford textbook of clinical pharmacology and drug therapy. Oxford University Press, Oxford

Gräsbeck R, Ahlström T (eds) (1981) Reference values in laboratory medicine. The current state of the art. Wiley, Chichester

Greenblatt DJ (1977) Reduced serum albumin concentration in the elderly: a report from the Boston collaborative drug surveillance program. J Am Geriatr Soc 27:20–22

Greenblatt DJ, Allen MD, Locniskar A, Harmatz JS, Shader RI (1979) Lorazepam kinetics in the elderly. Clin Pharmacol Ther 26:103–113

Greenblatt DJ, Divoll MK, Albernethy DR, Harmatz JS, Shader RI (1982a) Antipyrine kinetics in the elderly: prediction of age-related changes in benzodiazepine oxidizing capacity. J Pharmacol Exp Ther 220:120–126

Greenblatt DJ, Sellers EM, Shader RI (1982b) Drug disposition in old age. N Engl J Med 306:1081–1088

Greenblatt DJ, Divoll MK, Harmatz JS, Shader RI (1988) Antipyrine absorption and disposition in the elderly. Pharmacology 36:125–133

Greenblatt DJ, Harmatz JS, Shader RI (1991) Clinical pharmacokinetics of anxiolytics and hypnotics in the elderly. Therapeutic considerations. Clin Pharmacokinet 21 (3):165–177

Gribbin B, Pickering TG, Sleight P, Peto R (1971) Effect of age and high blood pressure on baroreflex sensitivity in man. Circ Res 29:424–431

Guarnieri T, Filburn CR, Zitnik G, Roth GS, Lakatta EG (1980) Contractile and biochemical correlates of beta-adrenergic stimulation of the aged heart. Am J Physiol 239H:501–508

Hagberg JM, Allen WK, Seals DR et al (1985) A hemodynamic comparision of young and older endurance athletes during exercise. J Appl Physiol 58:2041

Hainsworth R, Al-Shamma YMH (1988) Cardiovascular responses to upright tilting in healthy subjects. Clin Sci 74:17–22

Hale WE, Stewart RB, Marks RG (1983) Haematological and biochemical laboratory values in an ambulatory elderly population: an analyis of the effects of age, sex and drugs. Age Ageing 12:275–284

Haman D (1981) The aging process. Proc Natl Acad Sci USA 78 (11):7124

Hanger HC, Sainsbury R, Gilchrist NL, Beard MEJ (1991a) Erythrocyte sedimentation rates in the elderly: a community study. N Z Med J 104:134–136

Hanger HC, Sainsbury R, Gilchrist NL, Beard MEJ, Duncan JM (1991b) A community study of vitamin B12 and folate levels in the elderly. J Am Geriatr Soc 39:1155–1159

Harris EK (1988) Proposed goals for analytical precision and accuracy in single-point diagnostic testing. Theoretical basis and comparision with data from College of American Pathologists proficiency surveys. Arch Pathol Lab Med 112:416–420

Hayflick L (1961) The limited in vitro life-time of human diploid cell strains. Exp Cell Res 25:585

Hayflick L (1975) Current theories of biological aging. Fed Proc 34:9

Herd B, Wynne H, Wright P, James OFW, Woodhouse KW (1991) The effect of age on glucuronidation and sulphation in human liver. Br J Clin Pharmacol 32:768–770

Hollister LE (1981) General principles of treatng the elderly with drugs. In: Jarvic L (ed) Clinical pharmacology and the aged patient. Raven, New York, pp 1–9

Horn JL, Cattell RB (1967) Age differences in fluid and crystallized intelligence. Acta Psychol 26:107–129

Hultsch, D.F (1971) Organization and memory in adulthood. Hum Dev 14:16–29

Hunt CM, Westerkam WR, Stave GM, Wilson JA (1992) Hepatic cytochrome P-4503A (CYP3A) activity in the elderly. Mech Ageing Dev 64 (1-2):189–199

Inglis J (1962) Effects of age on responses to dichotic listening. Nature 194:1101

James GD, Sealey JE, Muller F, Alderman M, Madhavan S et al (1986) Renin relationship to sex, race and age in a normotensive population. J Hypertens 4 [Suppl 5]:387–389

Jernigan JA, Gudat JC, Blake JL, Bowen L, Lezotte DC (1980) Reference values for blood findings in relatively fit eldery persons. J Am Geriatr Soc 28 (7):308–314

Kafetz K (1984) Electrolytes, urea, creatinine and uric acid. In: Hodkinson M (ed) Clinical biochemistry in the elderly. Churchill Livingsone, Edinburgh, pp 170–171

Kato R, Takanaka A (1968) Metabolism of drugs in old rats. I. Activities of NADPH-linked election transport and drug-metabolising enzyme systems in liver microsomes of old rats. Jpn J Pharmacol 18:381–388

Kausler DH (1982) Experimental psychology and human aging. Wiley, New York

Kay H (1955) Some experiments on adult learning. 35th Long International Association of Gerontology, London 1954: old age in the modern world. Livingstone, Edingburgh, pp 259–267

Kelliher GJ, Conahan ST (1980) Changes in vagal activity and response to muscarinic receptor agonists with age. J Gerontol 45:842–849

Kelly A, Munan I, Clerc C, Plante G, Billon B (1979) Patterns of change in selected serum chemical parameters of middle and later years. J Gerontol 34:37–40

Kelly JG, McGarry K, O'Malley K, O'Brien ET (1982) Bioavailability of labetalol increases with age. Br J Clin Pharmacol 14:304–305

Kendall MJ, Woods KL, Wilkins MR, Worthington DJ (1982) Responsiveness to beta-adrenergic stimulation: the effects of age are cardioselective. Br J Clin Pharmacol 14:821–826

Kennedy HL, Horan MJ, Sprague MK, Padgett NE, Shriver KK (1983) Ambulatory blood pressure in healthy normotensive males. Am Heart J 106:717–722

Kennedy RD, Caird FI (1981) Physiology of aging of the heart. Cardiovasc Clin 12 (1):3

Kennedy RD, Andrews GR, Caird FI (1977) Ischemic heart disease in the elderly. Br Heart J 39:1121

Kenshalo DR (1977) Age changes in touch, vibration, temperature, kinesthesis and pain sensitivity. In: Birren JE, Schaie KW (eds) Handbook of the psychology of aging. Van Nostrand Reinhold, New York, pp 562–579

Klein C, Gerber JG, Gal J, Nies AS (1986) Beta-adrenergic receptors in the elderly are not less sensitive to timolol. Clin Pharmacol Ther 40:161–164

Klein C, Gerber JG, Payne NA, Nies AS (1990) The effect of age on the sensitivity of the α1-adrenoceptor to phenylephrine and prazosin. Clin Pharmacol Ther 47:535–539

Kohn R (1985) Heart and cardiovascular system. In: Finch CE, Schneider E (eds) Handbook of the biology of aging, 2nd edn. Van Nostrand Reinhold, New York

Kohn RR (1977) Heart and cardiovascular system. In: Finch C, Hayflick L (eds) Handbook of the biology in aging. New York, Van Nostrand Reinhold

Kopelman MD (1986) The cholinergic neurotransmitter system in human memory and dementia: a review. Q J Exp Psychol 38A:535–573

Kruger A (1987) The limits of normality in elderly patients. In: Hamblin JJ (ed) Ballieres clinical haematology. International practice and research, 1 (2). Balliere Tindall, London, pp 271–289

Lakatta E (1979) Alterations in the cardiovascular system that occur in advanced age. Fed Proc 38:163–167

Lakatta EG (1989) Arterial pressure and aging. Int J Cardiol 25:81–89

Lakatta EG, Yin FCP (1982) Myocardial aging: functional alterations and related cellular mechanisms. Am J Physiol 242:H927–941

Lamy PP (1986) Drug therapy in the elderly. Pharm Int 7:46–59

Lamy PP (1991) Physiological changes due to age. Pharmacodynamic changes of drug action and implications for therapy. Drugs Aging 1 (5):385–404

Lasagna L (1971) Influence of age on analgesic pain relief. J Am Med Assoc 218:1831

Lasagna L, Mosteller F, von Felsinger JM, Beecher HK (1954) A study of the placebo response. Am J Med 16:770–779

Leask RGS, Andrews GR, Caird FI (1973) Normal values for sixteen blood constituents in the elderly. Age Ageing 2:14–23

Levinson DJ et al (1978) The seasons of a man's life. Ballantine, New York

Lienert GA (1969) Testaufbau und Testanalyse, 3rd edn. Beltz, Weinheim

Lindeman RD (1992) Changes in renal function with aging. Implications for treatment. Drugs Aging 2 (5):423–431

Lindemann RD, Lee RD Jr, Yiengst MJ, Shock NW (1966) Influence of age, renal disease, hypertension, diuretics and calcium on the antidiuretic response to suboptimal infusions of vasopressin. J Lab Clin Med 68:206–223

Lindemann RD, Tobin J, Shock NW (1985) Longitudinal studies on the rate of decline in renal function with age. J Am Geriatr Soc 33:278–285

Lindenfeld J, Groves BM (1982) Cardiovascular function and disease in the aged. In: Schrier RW (ed) Clinical medicine in the aged. Saunders, Philadephia

Lipsitz LA (1989) Altered blood pressure homeostasis in advanced age: clinical and research implications. J Gerontol Med Sci 44 (6):M179–183

Manyari DE, Patterson C, Johnson D, Melendez L, Kostuk WJ, Cape RDT (1990) Atrial and ventricular arrhythmias in asymptomatic active elderly subjects: correlation with left atrial size and left ventriclar mass. Am Heart J 119:1069–1076

Manz M, Mletzko R, Jung W, Luederitz B (1990) Neue Aspekte zum klinischen Einsatz von Antiarrhythmika unter besonderer Berücksichtigung der Akuttherapie ventrikulärer Tachykardien (Lidocain vs. Ajmalin). [New aspects of the clinical use of anti-arrhythmia agents with special reference to acute therapy of ventricular tachycardia (lidocaine vs. ajmaline).] Herz 15 (2):79–89

Marchesini G, Bianchi GP, Fabritt E et al (1990) Synthesis of urea after a protein-rich meal in normal man in relation to ageing. Age Ageing 10:4–10

Marcus DL, Shadick N, Crantz J et al (1987) Low serum B12 levels in a hematologically normal elderly subpopulation. J Am Geriatr Soc 35:635–638

Marsh GR, Thompson LW (1977) Psychophysiology of aging. In: Birren JE, Schaie KW (eds) Handbook of the psychology of aging. Van Nostrand Reinhold, New York, pp 219–248

Martin CJ, Das S, Young AC (1979) Measurement of the dead space volume. J Appl Physiol 47:319–324

Matejcek M (1984) Elektroenzephalogramm (EEG). In: Oswald WD, Herrmann WM, Kanowski S, Lehr UM, Thomae H (eds) Gerontologie: Medizinische, psychologische und sozialwissenschaftliche Grundbegriffe. Kohlhammer, Stuttgart, pp 69–77

Mattila KS, Kuusela V, Pelliniemi TT et al (1986) Haematological laboratory findings in the elderly: influence of age and sex. Scand J Clin Lab Invest 46:411–415

McAdam W, Robinson RA (1956) Senile intellectual deterioration and the electroencephalogram. J Ment Sci 103:819–825

McDaniel G (1992) Biophysical changes of the older adult. In: Bullock BL, Philbrook Rosenthal P (eds) Pathophysiology: adaptions and alterations in function, 3rd edn. Lippincott, Philadelphia, pp 156–176

McLean KA, ONeill PA, Davies I (1989) Are the elderly dehydrated? A study to determine plasma osmolality in a community population. Clin Sci 77 (21):7

McMartin DN, OConnor JA, Fasco MJ, Kaminsky LS (1980) Influence of ageing and induction of rat liver and kidney microsomal mixed function oxidase systems. Toxicol Appl Pharmacol 54:411–419

Medvedev ZA (1972) Repetition of molecular-genetic information as a possible factor in evolutionary changes of life-span. Exp Gerontol 7:124

Melamed E, Lavy S, Bentin S, Cooper G, Rinot Y (1980) Reduction in regional cerebral blood flow during normal aging in man. Stroke 11:410–416

Michelsen S, Otterstad JE (1990) Blood pressure response during maximal exercise in apparently healthy men and women. J Intern Med 227:157–163

Milne JS, Wiliamson J (1972) Erythrocyte sedimentation rate in older people. Geront Clin 14:36–42

Morgenstern N, Byyny RL (1992) Epidemiology of hypertension in the elderly. Drugs Aging 2 (3):222–242

Mulkerrin EC, Arnold JD, Dewar R, Sykes D, Rees A, Pathy MS (1992) Glycosylated haemoglobin in the diagnosis of diabetes mellitus in elderly people. Age Ageing 21 (3):175–177

Mundy-Castle AC, Hurst LA, Beerstecher DM, Prinsloo T (1954) The electroencephalogram in the senile psychoses. Electroencephalogr Clin Neurophysiol 6:245–252

Myers J, Froelicher VF (1990) Optimizing the exercise test for pharmacological investigators. Circulation 82:1839–1846

Nation RL, Triggs EJ, Selig M (1977) Lignocaine kinetics in cardiac patients and aged subjects. Br J Clin Pharmacol 4:439–448

Nicolau GY, Haus E (1989) Chronobiologic reference values in clinical chemistry. Endocrinologie 27 (4):197–230

Nicolau GY, Haus E, Lakatua DJ, Bogdan C, Sacett-Lundeen L, Popescu M, Petrescu E, Robu E, Reilly C (1986) Circannual rhythms of laboratory parameters in serum of elderly subjects. Evaluation by cosinor analysis. Endocrinologie 24 (4):281–292

Novak LP (1972) Aging, total body potassium, fat-free mass and cell mass in males and females between 18 and 85. J Gerontol 27:438–444

O'Brien E, Murphy J, Tyndall A, Atkins N, Mee F, McCarthy G, Staessen J, Cox J, O'Malley K (1991) Twenty-four-hour ambulatory blood pressure in men and women aged 17 to 80 years: the Allied Irish Bank Study. J Hypertens 9:355–360

O'Malley K, Kelly JC, Swift CG (1987) Responsiveness to drugs. In: Swift CG (ed) Clinical pharmacology in the elderly. Dekker, New York, pp 83–101

Obrist WD (1979) Electroencephalographic changes in normal aging and dementia. In: Hoffmeister H, MÅller H (eds) Brain function in old age. Springer, Berlin Heidelberg New York, pp 102–111

Oswald WD, Fleischmann UM (1985) Psychometrics in gerontological research: models, methods and results. In: Bergener M, Ermini M, Stähelin HB (eds) Tresholds in aging. Academic, London, pp 384–420

Overstall PW (1982) Benzodiazepines, sleep and daytime performance. Medicine Publishing Foundation, Oxford, pp 15–19 (Medicine symposium no 10)

Palm D, Wiemer G (1982) Alter, Rezeptoren und Neurotransmitter. In: Bente D, Coper H, Kanowski S (eds) Hirnorganische Psychosyndrome im Alter. Springer, Berlin Heidelberg New York, pp 162–175

Palmer GJ, Ziegler MG, Lake CR (1978) Response of norepinephrine and blood pressure to stress increases with age. J Gerontol 33:482–487

Perry EK, Gibson PH, Blessed G, Perry RH, Tomlinson BE (1977) Neurotransmitter enzyme abnormalities in senile dementia: choline acetyltransferase and glutaminic and decarboxylase activities in neocropsy brain tissue. J Neurosci 34:247–265

Pfefferbaum A, Ford JM, Wenegrat B, Tinklenberg JR, Kopell BS (1982) Electrophysiological approaches to the study of aging and dementia. In: Corkin S, Davis KL, Growdon JH, Usdin H, Wurtman RJ (eds) Alzheimer's disease: a report of progress in research. Raven, New York, pp 83–91

Phillips PA, Rolls BJ, Ledingham JJG, Forsling ML, Morton JJ et al (1984) Reduced thirst after water deprivation in healthy elderly men. N Engl J Med 311:753–759

Pickering G (1968) High blood pressure. Churchill Livingstone, London

Piha SJ (1991) Cardiovascular autonomic reflex tests: normal responses and age-related reference values. Clin Physiol 11:277–290

Poon LW (1985) Differences in human memory with aging. In: Birren JE, Schaie KW (eds) Handbook of the psychology of aging, 2nd edn. Van Nostrand Reinhold, New York, pp 427–462

Port S, Cobb F, Colema E, Jones RH (1980) Effect of age on the response of the left ventricular ejection fraction to exercise. N Engl J Med 303:1133

Posner J, Danhjof M, Teunissen MWE, Breimer DD, Whiteman PD (1987) The disposition of antipyrine and its metabolites in young and elderly healthy volunteers. Br J Clin Pharmacol 24:51–55

Proper R, Wall F (1972) Left ventricular stroke volume measurements not affected by chronologic aging. Am Heart J 83:843

Queralt¢ JM, Boyd JC, Harris EK (1993) On the calculation of reference change values, with examples from a long-term study. Clin Chem 39 (7):1398–1403

Rabbit P (1965) Changes in problem solving ability in old age. In: Birren JE, Schaie KW (eds) Handbook of the psychology of aging. Van Nostrand Reinhold, New York, pp 606–625

Rabbit P (1986) An age-decrement in the ability to ignore irrelevant information. J Gerontol 20:233–238

Rapoport SI, Duara R, London ED, Margolin RA, Schwartz M, Cutler NE, Partanen M, Shinohara NL (1983) Glucose metabolism of the aging nervous system. In: Samuel D, Algeri S, Gershon S, Grimm VE, Toffano G (eds) Aging of the brain. Raven, New York, pp 111–121

Rechtschaffen A, Kales A (1968) A manual for standardized terminology, techniques and scoring system for sleep stages of human subjects. Public Health Service, US Government Printing Office, Washington DC

Reidenberg MM, Levy M, Warner H, Coutinho CB, Schartz MA et al (1978) Relationship between diazepam and dose, plasma level, age, and central nervous system depression. Clin Pharmacol Ther 23:371–374

Robertson DRC, Waller DG, Renwick AG, George CF (1988) Age-related changes in the pharmacokinetics and pharmacodynamics of nifedipine. Br J Clin Pharmacol 25:297–305

Rodeheffer RJ, Gerstenblith G, Becker LC, Fleg JL, Weisfeldt ML, Lakatta EG (1984) Exercise cardiac output is maintained with advancing age in healthy human subjects: cardiac dilatation and increased stroke volume compensate for a diminished heart rate. Circulation 69:203–213

Rogers H, Spector R (1984) Aids to Clinical pharmacology and therapeutics. Churchill Livingstone, Edinburgh

Roth GS (1980) Age-associated changes in hormone action: the role of receptors. In: Schimke RT (ed) Biological mechanisms in aging. United States Department of Health and Human Services, Washington DC, p 678

Roth GS, Hess GD (1982) Changes in the mechanisms of hormone and neurotransmitter action during aging: current status of the role of receptor and postreceptor alterations. Mech Ageing Dev 20:175–194

Roubicek J, Roth Z (1967) EEG frequency analysis related to age in normal adults. Electroencephalogr Clin Neurophysiol 23:162–167

Rowe JW, Troen BR (1980) Sympathetic nervous system and aging in man. Endocrinol Rev 1 (2):167–179

Rowe JW, Andres R, Tobin JD, Shock NW (1976) The effect of age on creatinine clearance in men: a cross-sectional and longitudinal study. J Gerontol 31:155–163

Rubin PC, Scott PJW, Mc Lean K, Reid JL (1982) Plasma noradrenaline and clearance in relation to age and blood pressure in man. Eur J Clin Invest 12:121–125

Saar N, Gordon RD (1979) Variability of plasma catecholamine levels: age, duration of posture and time of day. Br J Clin Pharmacol 8:353–358

Salthouse TA, Somberg BL (1982) Isolating the age deficit in speeded performance. J Gerontol 37:59–63

Santrock JW (1985) Adult devolopment and aging. Brown, Dubuque

Scarpace P, Tumer N, Mader L (1991) β-Adrenergic function in aging: basic mechanisms and clinical implication. Drug Aging 1:116–129

Schimke RT (ed) (1980) Biological mechanisms in aging. United States Department of Health and Human Services, Washington DC

Schlant RC, Friesinger GC, Leonard JJ (1990) Clinical competence in exercise testing. A statement for physicians from the ACP/ACC/AHA task force on clinical privileges in cardiology. Circulation 83:1884–1888

Schmidtke H (1951) öber die Messung der psychischen ErmÅdung mit Hilfe des Flimmertests. Psychol Forsch 23:409–463

Schmucker DL, Woodhouse KW, Wang RK, Wynne H, James OFW et al (1990) Effect of age and gender on in vitro properties of human liver microsomal monooxygenases. Clin Pharmacol Ther 48:365–374

Schocken DD, Roth GS (1977) Reduced beta-adrenergic receptor concentrations in aging man. Nature 267:856

Scott JC, Stanski DR (1987) Decreased fentanyl and alfentanil dose requirements with age. A simultaneous pharmacokinetic and pharmacodynamic evaluation. J Pharmacol Exp Ther 240:159–166

Scott PJW, Hosie J, Scott MGB (1988) A double-blind and cross-over comparison of once daily doxazosin and placebo with steady-state pharmacokinetics in elderly hypertensive patients. Br J Clin Pharmacol 34:119–123

Shillinford SJ, Shillingford CA (1987) Aspects of pharmacokinetic and pharmacodynamic research in the elderly. In: Hindmarch I, Stonier PD (eds) Human psychopharmacology. Wiley, Chichester, pp 201–211

Shok NW, Watkin DM, Yiengest MJ et al (1963) Age differences in the water content of the body as related to basal oxygen consuption in males. J Gerontol 18:1–8

Sohal R, Allen R (1985) Relationship between metabolic rate, free radicals, differentiation and aging: a unified theory. In: Woodhead A, Blachett A, Hollaender A (eds) Molecular biology of aging. Plenum, New York

Sparrow D, Rowe JE, Silbert JE (1980) Cross sectional and longitudinal chenges in the reythrocyte sedimentation rate in men. J Gerontol 36:180–184

Spilker B (1986) Guide to clinical interpretation of data. Raven, New York

Squires K, Goodin D, Starr A (1979) Event-related potentials in development aging, and dementia. In: Lehmann D, Callaway E (eds) Human evoked potentials: applications and problems. Plenum, New York, pp 383–396

Stolarek I, Scott PJW, Caird FI (1991) Physoiological changes due to age Implications for cardiovascular drug therapy. Drugs Aging 1 (6):467–476

Swift CG, Homeida M, Halliwell M, Roberts CJC (1978) Antipyrine dispositin and liver size in the elderly. Eur J Clin Pharmacol 14:149–152

Swift CG, Haythorne JM, Clarke P, Stenvenson IH (1981) The effect of aging on measured responses to single doses of oral temazepam. Br J Clin Pharmacol 11:413–414

Tejada C, Strong JP, Montenegro MR et al (1968) Distribution of coronary and aortic atheroclerosis by geographic location, race and sex. Lab Invest 18:509

Thompson WL, Brunelle RL, Enas GG, Simpson PJ, Walker RL (1990) Routine laboratory tests in clinical trials. Supplemental tables – update 1990. Supplement to: Cato A.E. (ed) Clinical trials and tribulations. Dekker, New York (1988)

Thurlbeck WM, Angus GE (1975) Growth and aging of the normal human lung, Chest 67:38–78

Tietz NW, Wekstein DR, Shuey DF, Brauer GA (1984) A two-year longitudinal reference range study for selected serum encymes in a population more than 60 years of age. J.Am Geriatr Soc 32:563–570

Tietz NW, Shuey DF, Wekstein DR (1992) Laboratory values in fit aging individuals. Sexagenarians thrugh centenaarians. Clin Chem 38 (6):1167–1185

Tomlinson BE (1982) Plaques, tangles and Alzheimer's disease. Psychol Med 12:449–459

Tomlinson BE, Blessed A, Roth M (1968) Observations on the brains of non-demented old people. J Neurol Sci 7:331–356

Triggs EJ, Nation RL, Long A, Ashley JJ (1975) Pharmacokinetics in the elderly. Eur J Clin Pharmacol 8:55–62

Trowbridge EA, Reardon DM, Bradey J, Hutschinson D, Warren CW (1989) Automated haematology: construction of univariate reference ranges for blood cell count and size. Med Lab Sci 46:23–32

Tsujimoto G, Hashimoto K, Hoffman BB (1989a) Pharmacokinetic and pharmacodynamic principles of drug therapy in old age, part 1. Int J Clin Pharmacol Ther Toxicol 27 (1):13–26

Tsujimoto G, Hashimoto K, Hoffman BB (1989b) Pharmacokinetic and pharmacodynamic principles of drug therapy in old age, part 2. Int J Clin Pharmacol Ther Toxicol 27 (3):102–116

Van Brummelen P, Båhler FR, Kiowski W, Amann FW (1981) Age-related decrease in cardiac and peripheral vascular responsiveness to isoprenaline: Studies in normal subjects. Clin Sci (Oxf) 60:571–577

Vargas, E, Lye M, Faragher EB, Goddard C, Moser B, Davies J (1986) Cardiovascular haemodynamics and the response of vasopressin, aldosterone, plasma renin activity and plasma catecholamines to head-up tilt in young and old healthy subjects. Age Ageing 15:17–28

Veering BTH, Burm AGL, Souverijn JHM, Serree JMP, Spierdijk J (1990) The effect of age on serum concentrations of albumin α1-acid glycoprotein. Br J Clin Pharmacol 29:201–206

Vestal RE (1978) Drug use in the elderly – a review of problems and special considerations. Drugs 16:258-382

Vestal RE, Wood AJJ, Shand DG (1979a) Reduced β-adrenoceptor sensivity in the elderly. Clin Pharmacol Ther 26:181–186

Vestal RE, Wood AJJ, Branch RA, Shand DG, Wilkinson GR (1979b) Effects of age and cigarette smoking on propanolol disposition. Clin Pharmacol Ther 26:181–186

Vita G, Princi P, Calabro R, Toscano A, Manna L, Messina C (1986) Cardiovascular reflex tests. Assessment of age-adjusted normal range. J Neurol Sci 75:263–274

Vokonas PS, Kannel WB, Cupples LA (1988) Epidemiology and risk of hypertension in the elderly: the Framingham Study. J Hypertens 6 [Suppl 1]:3–9

Wang HS, Busse EW (1969) EEG of healthy old persons – a longitudinal study. I. Dominant background activity and occipital rhythm. J Gerontol 24:419–426

Warrington EK, Sanders HI (1971) The fate of old memories. Q J Exp Psychol 23:432–442

Waugh NC, Norman DA (1965) Primary memory. Psychol Rev 72:89–104

Wechsler D (1958) The measurement and appraisal of adult intelligence. Williams and Wilkins, Baltimore

Weidenhammer W, Engel R (1988) Psychometrie und Elektroenzephalographie bei gesunden Hochbetagten. Z Gerontopsychol Psychiatr 1:105–115

Weisfeldt ML, Lakatta EG, Gerstenblith G (1992) Aging and the heart. In: Braunwald E (ed) Heart disease. Saunders, Philadelphia, pp 1656–1669

Welford AT (1977) Motor performance. In: Birren JE, Schaie KW (eds) Handbook of the psychology of aging. Van Nostrand Reinhold, New York, pp 450–496

West DW, Ash KO (1984) Adult reference intervals for 12 chemistry analytes: influences of age and sex. Am J Clin Pathol 81:71–76

Weyer G (1992) Methodologische Überlegungen zur Bestimmung von Therapierespondern in Nootropikastudien. In: Oldigs-Kerber J, Leonard JP (eds) Pharmakopsychologie: experimentelle und klinische Aspekte. Fischer, Jena, pp 380–393

Williams FM, Mutch EM, Nicholson E, Wynne H, Wright P et al (1989a) Human liver and plasma aspirin esterase. J Pharm Pharmacol 41:401–409

Williams FM, Wynne H, Woodhouse KW, Rawlins MD (1989b) Plasma aspirin esterase: the influence of old age and frailty. Age Ageing 18:39–42

Wilson RS, Kaszniak AW (1986) Longitudinal changes: progressive idiopathic dementia. In: Poon LW, Davis KL, Eisdorfer C, Gurland BJ, Kaszniak AW, Thompson LW (eds) Clinical memory assessment in older adults. American Psychological Association, Washington DC, pp 285–293

Woo J, Swaminathan R (1991) Plasma osmolality in an elderly population. J Med 22 (2):69–75

Wood AJJ, Feely J (1985) Effect of age on sensitivity to drug. In: O'Mealey K (ed) Clinical pharmacology and drug treatment in the elderly. Churchill Livingstone, London, pp 39–51

Woodhouse KW, Wynne HA (1988) Age-related changes in liver size and hepatic blood flow: the influence on drug metabolism in the elderly. Clin Pharmaco-kinet 15:287–296

Woodhouse KW, Wynne HA (1992) Age-related changes in hepatic function. Implications for drug therapy. Drugs Aging 2 (3):243–255

Wynne HA, Cope LH, Mutch E, Rawlins MD, Woodhouse KW et al (1989) The effect of age upon liver volume and apparent liver blood flown healthy man. Hepatology 9:297–301

Wynne HA, Cope LH, Herd B, Rawlins MD, James OFW et al (1990a) The association of age and frailty with paracetamol conjugation in man. Age Ageing 19:419–424

Wynne HA, Goudouvenous J, Adams P, Rawlins MD, James OFW et al (1990b) Hepatic extraction of drugs: the effect of age using indocyanine green as a model substrate. Br J Clin Pharmacol 30:634–637

Yin FCP, Raizes GS, Guarnieri T et al (1978) Age asociated decrease in ventricular response to hemodynamic stress during beta-adrenergic blockade. Br Heart J 40:1349

Zauber NP, Zauber AG (1987) Hematologie data of healthy very old people. JAMA 257:2181–2184

Zaino EC (1981) Blood counts in the nonagenarian. N Y State J Med 8:1199–1200